THE RUNNING
FOOT DOCTOR

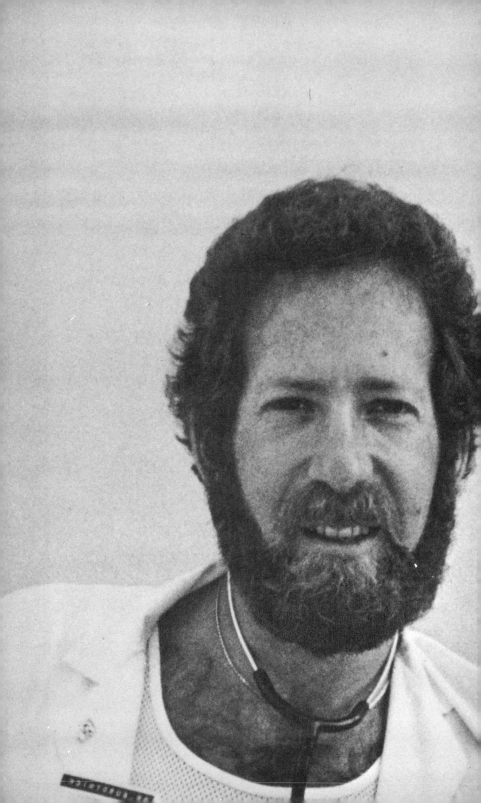

THE RUNNING FOOT DOCTOR

by
Steven I. Subotnick, D.P.M., M.S.

illustrated by
Stanley G. Newell, D.P.M.

Published by
WORLD PUBLICATIONS

Acknowledgements

Through my years of running and treating runners, I have had the opportunity to treat and meet many wonderful people. Sports medicine and, in particular, podiatric sports medicine has grown in leaps and bounds. We have learned from the opportunity to treat runners and get feedback from runners. I would, above all, like to thank them for their help.

I also thank Nancy Vierra for the fantastic job she did in helping to write this book, and the staff of *Runner's World*, Joe Henderson in particular, for the editing job. A great amount of work was done by Dr. Stan Newell, a sports medicine podiatrist in Seattle, who labored over the illustrations used in this book. Many of the illustrations were taken from my textbook on sports medicine by Futura Publications, which likewise were illustrated by Dr. Newell.

© 1977 by
WORLD PUBLICATIONS
P.O. Box 366, Mt. View, CA. 94042

*No information in this book may be reprinted in
any form without permission from the publisher.*

Library of Congress Catalog Number 77-73653
ISBN 0-89037-116-4 hardback
ISBN 0-89037-117-2 paperback
Second Printing, July 1977

This book is dedicated to my wife, Jan, and to my children, Markie, Ali and Kari.

Contents

Introduction

In May 1976, I met with Bob Anderson and Joe Henderson of *Runner's World* to discuss something that had formed in my mind several years earlier. This was a book for the running public—a book telling how I got interested in running, what I have learned as a runner and how I have been able to relate what I know as a podiatrist to sports medicine in general, running medicine in particular.

Anderson and Henderson thought it would be a good idea to have this book center around running, yet be broad enough to attract the interest of all forms of athletes. We thought this was fairly logical since running is the primary activity in almost all sports and since I had found that even swimmers have injuries similar to those of runners—muscle injuries or strains, for example.

Then I thought about the type of audience we were trying to reach. Basically, we were aiming at the type of patients I treat, yet my athlete patients range anywhere from junior high school students on up to the middle-aged or elderly joggers. How could I relate equally well to a student and to a business executive. This was going to be somewhat difficult, but the cohesive bond among them all was their interest in their sport, basically running.

The majority of my athletic patients are runners. But I also see race walkers, skiers, tennis buffs, gymnasts, football and basketball players, and participants in field hockey, soccer and various forms of field events (high jump, discus and so on). I also see golfers and bowlers as well as non-athletes for basic foot care. These people are not runners but of course all of them walk. I apply treatment principles used with the general public to runners as well as applying what I know about running to my less active patients.

I concluded that, since running is a basic activity of most sports, I could tie everything together by covering injuries I see in running. I could explain about aches and pains that occur during running and how athletes can roughly tell what may be wrong with themselves. I could give them information for deciding what they may need to do to prevent getting injured more seriously, what they might have to do to rehabilitate themselves and when it is necessary to seek help from a medical specialist such as a sports podiatrist.

Henderson had a good idea for putting this information across. He said, "Tell stories."

"What do you mean, tell stories?" I said.

He said, "Tell about your start in podiatry, your start in sports medicine, your start in running, about your patients, your successes and failures, and what you have learned in the past few years. Obviously, when you began not much had been written about the podiatrist in sports, and not much was known. Your role in sports medicine has evolved over the past few years. Wouldn't it be interesting to talk about its evolution, about where it has gone and where you think it might go?"

I said, "Sure, I think that's great! But do you think anyone would be interested in how I got started and what my thoughts are?"

Henderson answered, "Certainly. Readers relate easier to stories about people like themselves than to abstract scientific discussions."

He was suggesting a book about running and how I related to my patients. I said, "Great! This is what I really wanted to do in the first place, but I didn't think anyone would want to read it."

When I first started working in sports medicine about five years ago, I kept thinking how great it would be if I could someday write a book that all my patients could read. I could say, "Go to Chapter Four and read this. This is about the same type of problem you have. See what you think." This would help me, and it might help thousands of runners who might never have the chance to see someone interested in running.

I recently wrote a textbook on sports medicine which is for the doctor, or the interested coach or trainer. This is a more scientific book and does not "tell stories," but it is filled with information. My job here is to put this information into a more interesting form so that the book flows, informs and excites the runner-reader.

Steven I. Subotnick, D.P.M., M.S.
Hayward, Calif.
December 1976

Left foot, right foot, wet foot, dry foot
Low foot, high foot, slow foot, quick foot.

Trick feet, sick feet, up feet, down feet,
small feet, big feet.

Feet in the morning, feet at night.
How many, many feet I meet.

Foot Book, Dr. Seuss

part I

TAKING PODIATRY PERSONALLY

1

Foot Doctoring

While at Lewis and Clark College in Oregon, I played one year of football and realized that small people get hurt in that sport. I then skied competitively for five years. During the summers, I life-guarded. I recall enjoying running about three miles a day up and down the beaches. But I never knew that running was meant to be an everyday activity. It just felt good.

One summer, I was teaching swimming to a podiatrist's children. Dr. Henry Swearingen asked me what I was going to do with my life.

I said, "I really don't know, but I thought I might like to become a professor, teach medical school or become a doctor."

"Why don't you investigate the field of podiatry?" was his reply. We went to his office, talked together and it didn't take me long to decide that this was just what I wanted to do—get involved in a field where I could become a specialist.

Somehow, I got through four years at the California College of Podiatric Medicine in San Francisco, a year of internship and another year of residency, accepted a teaching position and established a private practice—plus starting a family. There wasn't much time to think about, let alone practice, sports during those years.

Then one day another podiatrist, Dr. Tom Sgarlato asked me what I knew about skiing. I said I knew a fair amount, since I had raced for about five years.

He continued, "What do you know about the function of

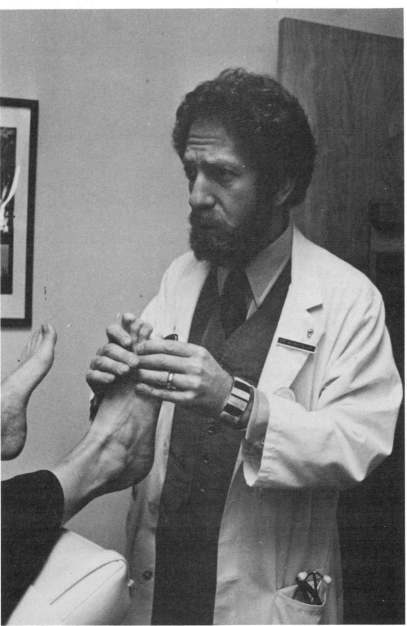

A background in sports indirectly led Dr. Subotnick into podiatry, and his work with runners' feet led him to run himself.

skiing, about the biomechanics of skiing, about the science of motion of skiing?"

I said to myself, "Well, not a whole lot, but that shouldn't be too hard to figure out. I am getting ready to teach biomechanics and I know how to ski."

I thought about this for a long time and then did some experiments. I went to the mountains with a small group of test subjects, and observed functional changes on the hills as they wore various foot supports and wedges. I concluded that I could signficantly improve skiing by using these devices. I came to a further conclusion that many people have deformities of the lower extremities which really make it difficult (if not impossible) to "set an edge" while skiing on a flat base. I subsequently published a paper on my findings, which basically was ignored until recently. (Now, I understand that it is widely used by people who teach skiing.)

This was the sum of my sports background when I received a fateful phone call from Bob Lualhati, track coach at Skyline College near San Francisco. He asked what I could do to help his cross-country team's injuries.

Since I really did not know what I was going to find, I suggested that the best approach would be for me to examine the entire team and treat the runners as necessary, at no charge. All of us working together might learn something that would be of benefit to athletes everywhere.

Six or seven cross-country runners had problems ranging from achilles tendonitis, to pain about the knee, to arch pain. One of them had recurring stress fractures.

Basic facts were realized immediately during preliminary examinations. All of the runners were extremely tight in the muscles of the backs of their legs. These muscles are called the "gravity" muscles, and they are the primary movers at toe-off. (The "anti-gravity" muscles are in the front of the legs, and they decelerate the foot as it contacts the ground.)

You could almost identify them as runners from across the room, as they walked, because of this tightness. This tightness, and a strength imbalance between muscles in the back of the legs (strong) and front (weak) contributed to shin splints, heel cord strain and injuries to the foot.

I also found that most of these runners appeared to have rather narrow ranges of motion in the major joint of the foot, the subtalar. They had much less motion than the normal non-running population.

I found that the majority of the runners appeared to contact a little bit more on the outside of their feet than the average person. This was also demonstrated by excessive wear on the outside of the heels of their shoes.

And finally, I noted that most of the runners really did not have any serious or advanced foot deformity based on standards for a less active group. Most had fairly good structure with only minor imbalances.

It became apparent to me that for everyday activities this group would generally have no foot-related problems. Running, however, appeared to require almost perfect structure and function. I then came to realize that what I needed to do was provide for better function with some form of foot support.

Various types of supports, "orthotics," would be needed for various activities. The plastic orthotics I used for the general public would, with some modifications, be just fine for the runner's everyday activities as well as long, slow distance training. But a softer, more flexible support would be necessary for short, fast training and racing.

I made both types of orthotics for the Skyline College team. And I placed all the runners on exercises for stretching the tight, strong muscles and strengthening the weak muscles.

As I watched my patients run, I noticed that invariably one foot either turned in or turned out more than the other foot. One leg rotated more or less than the other leg. It became apparent that no one was perfect in his running stride, at least nobody I had seen.

When I placed the runners in the softer supports, less wobbling took place in the foot and they appeared to be in better balance. When I placed them in the plastic supports, dramatic changes were seen. Runners, who had run with their feet thrown to the side started lining their feet up straight ahead. Runners who had excessively bouncy gaits appeared to be smoother, and those who had sloppy toe-offs appeared to be stronger.

The runners said they noticed a great difference, and that they were running more efficiently and with less pain. When I treated people who complained of arch pain or pain in the achilles, they came back saying that their knees felt better, too. One runner's hip and back stopped hurting. So, it became apparent that I was helping the entire lower extremity of the runners.

Dr. George Sheehan was right—the foot must be the weak link in the runner suffering from an overuse injury. A new approach was needed—treating the cause, not the symptoms of an injury. The podiatrist's job would be to prevent those overuse injuries attributed to poor foot function.

Man without motion, self-movement, is society's failure.

2

A New Runner

I wrote to *Runner's World* about the work I had done with the Skyline College cross-country team. I remember saying, "I think I may be on to something that you might be interested in."

Joe Henderson was extremely interested. We met at my office, where I examined and treated Joe himself. He had been injured for several months and could do little running. He ran better with orthotics. He began to stretch, but his injured heel eventually required surgery.

At about the same time, Peter Stein, a local runner came into my office on Henderson's recommendation. Stein had very bad knee pain, but was hopeful that I would be able to cure him for the Boston Marathon two months later. I examined Peter and came to the conclusion that he had excessive flattening of the arch ("pronation") during weight-bearing, the time the arch should be a more rigid supportive structure. When the arch is excessively low, it is necessary for the leg to internally rotate. This causes a chain of events which may lead to overuse injury.

It became evident in Peter's case that the weak link in his running was the foot itself. Despite the fact that everything else was strong in his body, this imbalance or overpronation in the foot was always going to cause him a problem. I examined his knee carefully and could find only a tenderness underneath the kneecap and a "crunchy" feeling beneath the kneecap. This fit well into the diagnosis of chondromalacia of the patella, which is a common running injury.

I made soft orthotics for Stein and then rigid orthotics. For the first week or so, he was still extremely sore and had a great deal of trouble walking or jogging. We both were depressed, and I had almost come to the conclusion that my theories and diagnosis were wrong. Then, something happened.

Peter noticed the knee immediately responded to the harder, more rigid orthotics with the heel-stabilizing device. He began running longer and with decreasing pain. Two months later, he went to the Boston Marathon, where he wore his plastic supports throughout the race and had no pain whatsoever.

I also had him work on exercises to build up his quadriceps muscles, which appeared to be necessary to help stabilize his kneecap. I told Peter my thoughts about stretching before and after running.

We became very good friends, and Peter's project became making a runner of me. I recall vividly how he would advise my office staff to block out two-hour sessions in the afternoon so that we could run. He did this two or three times a week. He also would come visit on the weekends and run with me.

Stein and Bob Garnero came to the office one day for their treatment, then we went to my house for a run. I have a three-quarter-mile loop there. I ran around this twice, almost passed out from exhaustion and came home to shower and wait for their return after three or more laps.

We all sat down for lunch and Peter explained to my wife, Jan, how running before a meal really cuts down your appetite and helps you lose weight. Great, I thought. I weighed about 185 pounds and needed to lose 20-30. I had been relatively inactive for the past two years.

Peter then sat down, ate five sandwiches and had two glasses of milk. I couldn't believe it. I said to myself, "If this is how I am going to lose weight, I had better find another sport."

Stein, we later learned, is a big eater. He is one of the few people I know who can eat a full meal at home, and then come over and eat another dinner at my house.

I had run for about a week when Peter decided that it was time for me to do my first race. I packed my wife and kids into the station wagon and headed for a *Runner's World*-sponsored fun-run. This was a three-mile run.

I showed up in my Cost-Plus tennis shoes, a pair of old tennis shorts with ripped pockets and a dirty T-shirt. I lined up at the start with all the other runners. There was a great feeling there. Excitement was in the air. I was ready for the race of my life.

We started. I jogged along towards the front of the group for 30-40 seconds before I got a little bit tired. People began passing me. I figured I would just take it easy and it would really be no problem at all, because I had been a great jock in college.

I was almost dead last at the turnaround point and I recall the utter depression of realizing that this was only half of the race and that I would have to run all the way back. Joe Henderson's wife, Janet, was at the point and encouraged me so that I could finish before dark. My time was 29 minutes.

I obviously have progressed from there. Several months later, I ran the San Francisco Bay-to-Breakers race (about eight miles) in 64 minutes. One year after I started running, I finished a marathon in 3:39. Since then, I have run several other marathons, including Boston with my best time of 3:17.

Running has become a real part of my life, and I try to dedicate an hour a day to it. I race in local events. I am not the least embarrassed with slow performances. I love runners and associating with them, and we have learned from each other.

3

Self-Treatment

The next logical step after running my first fun-run was to prepare for the Bay-to-Breakers. I worked up from three to eight miles a day in two weeks—and experienced my first serious running injury.

Although I could barely walk, this injury was not going to stop me from running, so I taped up my leg and drove over to San Francisco for the famed race. The result was a pulled leg muscle which laid me up for two months. I could barely walk after the race, but I knew I was hooked. I had to run or do something. I had lost about 20-25 pounds and never felt better in my life.

So, shortly after the Bay-to-Breakers, I told *RW* publisher Bob Anderson of my plight. He suggested that I get a good bike and start working out on it. (I had been riding a bike for about the past week, but it was quite old and used.)

Bob and I drove to a bike shop and I shelled out $150 for a touring bike. I must have really been crazy in those early days, but I knew that I had to keep going.

This attitude, I see in retrospect, caused my first and most serious injury. Even now, it will plague me occasionally if I am not careful. Here is how it happened. (Ever notice how we runners love to talk about our injuries? Reminds me of my older patients who love to talk about their past operations.)

There is a large 1 1/2 mile hill behind my house which levels off to gentle, rolling hills and makes about a 10-mile loop if I

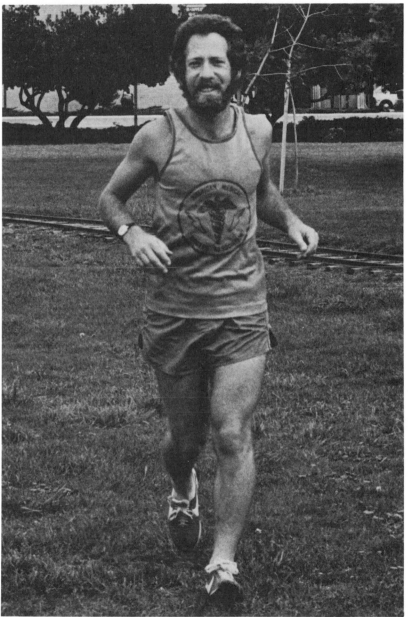

Subotnick the runner: His own injuries "have given me insights I never would have had as a non-running podiatrist."

travel the entire distance. I had been eyeing this hill for about a month after I started running, hoping that someday I would be strong enough to run it. One day I did just that. I looked up the hill, said I was ready and ran it.

I charged up the hill, turned around and started back down. On the way back, I noticed that something was wrong with my leg. I was so thrilled, this really did not matter. I just kept on running down the hill as fast as I could.

At the end of my run, I was almost limping, but it still didn't matter. I didn't stretch. I didn't cool down. I just got in the car with my family and went to the swimming pool. At the pool, my leg hurt and I knew something was wrong, but I figured it would go away soon. It didn't. The back of my leg, just below the knee, was somewhat swollen and extremely sore.

I had, basically, torn muscle fibers in the back of my leg due to my stupidity and anxiousness to be a good runner. And I had learned a lesson which will stay with me for the rest of my running career.

There have been other injuries. (They may be inevitable among runners, even among running doctors.) And while they have been unpleasant when they occurred, they have given me insights into sports medicine which I never would have had as a non-running podiatrist.

My good friend Dr. George Sheehan once told me that he learned more from his own injuries than from anything else. This is why a running doctor is so valuable. If he has run long enough, he probably has had the injury which his patients have or knows a number of people who have had it. And probably he also knows the practical instead of merely the theoretical solution to the trouble.

4

Travels with Tracy

Dennis Tracy is the thoroughbred—a race horse *extraordinaire.* He runs with rather short, choppy strides. He wastes no energy. He is experienced, knows all the tricks and likes to win.

One day, as I was jogging around the three-quarter-mile loop near my house, I noticed this rather slender fellow walking two Afghan hounds. He was wearing running shoes and jogging up and down. I sized him up as just another dog walker in fancy shoes.

A couple of days later, I was out again and saw this same fellow. This time he was running—about twice as fast as I, in the opposite direction. I turned around, somehow caught up to him and began talking.

I said, "Did you happen to run the Bay-to-Breakers this year?"

"Oh yeah," he said. "I've been running it for the past several years."

"I did pretty well this year—about 64 minutes," I bragged. "This was my first big race."

"I...uh...placed in the top 20 this year," he told me.

That blew me right out of the saddle. I later learned that Dennis is a 4:11 miler and probably can hold five-minute mile pace longer than almost anyone else in the area. He is a great runner, a natural.

We became good friends, and he decided he could convert me from a jogger to a runner. We ran together for about two years, religiously. He helped me get ready for the Avenue of the Giants Marathon by going on 13-14-mile runs on the weekends. We ran 6-8-mile fartlek-type workouts in the evenings, racing each other around the three-quarter mile loop. I later learned that he didn't get much good out of this because I was too slow for him, but he stayed with me.

One summer day, after I'd eaten five hot dogs and had two beers, Dennis decided it was time to give me a workout. He placed a 10-pound weight vest on me, took out his stop watch, and we ran up and down hills for about a half-hour. I suggested that I was going to throw up, and he nodded and said that this was good because it was going to make me tough.

"You have to be tough," he told me. "You have to be real tough. You have to hurt if you're going to win. It's not easy to be good, and it's even harder to be great."

Dennis talked to me about racing tactics, hill running and intervals. I got better, and ran faster and longer. Then things started to get away from me. I reached a point where I just wanted to run easy, no more fast stuff, no more hurting. I wasn't cut out to be that type of runner. I wasn't a thoroughbred.

So, I slowed down, way down. I re-evaluated myself and what running meant to me. Running had been too important, and I decided to make it part of a more balanced life. It gained a broader perspective—that of longevity. I realized you can't make a race horse out of a trotter, and at the very best I was a trotter.

Through Dennis I also came to realize that even race horses have their problems. He is not only a friend but a patient of mine, and I have treated him for a strain around his knee and around his kneecap. He also has recurring pain from a bump at the back of the heel.

When I examined Dennis several years ago, I found that he had a rather narrow range of motion and pretty good foot structure. In fact, he had almost the perfect arch, which flattened out only moderately when he ran. We took movies of him running and found that he is a toe runner. He has a tendency to shuffle along on the balls of his foot. Only when he is running quite slowly does his heel rock back and touch the surface. His heel has a tendency to slide up and down in his running shoe, and his weight tends to remain on the outside of his foot.

This rocking up and down and having the weight mostly on the outside of the foot probably are the main factors causing his heel bump. X-rays also showed he has an inherited shelf of bone which protrudes under the attachment of the achilles tendon. This naturally predisposes him to injury in this area.

It would be easier to treat Dennis if he had a flatter foot with more flexibility and more motion. But he doesn't. His foot functions with such a narrow range that it was very difficult to build any type of support for him which is comfortable. Yet he appeared to need some form of foot support for his heel problem.

We made supports which were semi-flexible, allowed him to run fast and yet somewhat supported his heel. This has helped him to such an extent that he has not needed any surgery, but if he is not careful he still gets a flare-up on the back of his heel.

The pain he has around the knee is somewhat of a mystery, for most of the knee pain I have seen has to do with the kneecap or with a strain to the outside of the knee from a tight iliotibial band. These problems tend to respond fairly well to foot supports and proper exercises for flexibility and to build up the muscles in the front of the thigh which stabilize the kneecap.

Dennis did all these exercises, has the foot supports (in fact, even has plastic supports for long-distance running and everyday use) and still has knee pain. He runs so fast, and is on the balls of his feet so much of the time, that the best supports in the world do not seem to help him.

The only support that is really effective when a runner is on the ball of his foot is a support which is under the ball. This must be flexible and soft so he can get on the ball of his foot in the first place. A plastic support can't go under the ball of the foot and still be comfortable or bend enough to allow you even to run at all.

Dennis has a problem, and so do all the other ball-of-the-foot runners who have overuse injuries. The only thing that will really help is a soft, flexible support and perhaps taping of the foot or else slowing down and letting the injuries heal up. Dennis Tracy does not like to slow down for anything, not even an injury.

Recently, I dropped out of a marathon after 22 miles and realized I had not been training hard enough. There was nothing else to do but call Tracy and ask him how to go about becoming a better runner. He was quick to point out that I had gained weight, looked sloppy and resembled a pig from the back when I was running. He also noted that I had no speed and that running long, slow distances would make me a long, slow runner. After not finishing the marathon, I wasn't even sure I could run long.

We began a program of interval training. I ran 220 yards close to all-out, followed by a 220 jog. I also did 440 repeats, 330 repeats and 110 sprints on the grass. Dennis and I would run the 2 ½ -3 miles from our homes to the local college track, work out on the track for approximately two miles, then run back uphill to our homes again.

This change in training taught me first that the only way to increase your speed is to run fast. Then it taught me that the way to increase your distance is to run farther. I noted that there are changes in your body after speed training which you just cannot get from distance training.

Dennis taught me that the long runs are basically to relax your muscles and allow you to recover from your interval training. He also noted that I should be doing interval training at least three times a week.

I looked around at the great runners and they all seemed to be doing intervals and improving because of this. I have no real desire to become a great runner, but I would like to improve. My long, slow distance running had been pleasant but I had become stale. Staleness in running demands a change, and that change for me appeared to be intervals.

While I will never be a thoroughbred runner, that didn't mean I couldn't learn from one.

part II

WHY WE GET HURT

5

How We Work

Biomechanics is the biology of motion, the study of mechanisms of movement. A biomechanical approach to injury is one which seeks out causes, corrects the causes and, we hope, stops the injury from recurring.

If the damage has been done from an injury, a biomechanical approach should reverse the process and the injury should go away. There are times, however, when the damage has progressed to the point that biomechanical control can't reverse it. In these cases, there has been enough rearrangement of soft tissue in the form of scar tissue that it is very difficult to stretch this tissue out and allow for normal function. We see this occasionally in severe tendonitis.

A biomechanical approach also may prevent injury from occurring. An example of this is someone who is just beginning to run, and has a rather weak foot structure. Preventive medicine would be to provide some form of support for the feet, while also encouraging the proper strengthening and flexibility exercises.

A biomechanical approach is somewhat "holistic" in that the entire patient, his running activities or other athletic activities and functionings must be looked into. Thus, the biomechanical approach we podiatrists use includes suggestions as to proper training and conditioning exercises as well as function.

What are proper biomechanics and proper function? To understand the whole, one has to divide the various phases of motion into smaller phases and study these.

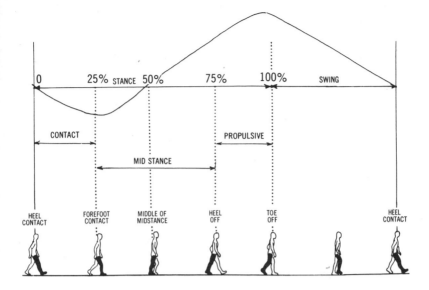

FIGURE 1

The Gait Cycle in Walking

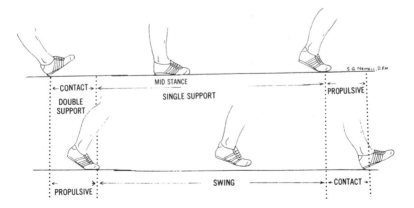

FIGURE 2

Coordinated Gait Cycles of Both Legs

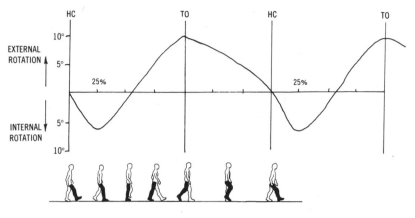

FIGURE 3

Rotations of the Leg and Effects on the Foot

We start with walking (*Figure 1*) and build into running. During walking, one foot is always on the ground in the "stance phase." The foot moving through the air is in "swing phase." (*Figure 2*).

The swing-phase foot is always associated with the leg which is internally rotated (*Figures 3 and 4*). This internal rotation takes place during swing and as the foot contacts the ground. The rotation then reverses itself, and external rotation begins.

Internal rotation is synonymous with the foot becoming flattened at contact. When the foot is on the ground and side-to-side motion is prevented, the kneecap faces in and the arch is lowered. We call this "pronation." This motion is necessary to have your foot act as a mobile adapter to varying types of surfaces.

The foot must be a mobile adapter at contact, but it quickly must become a rigid lever for a stable lift-off. As external rotation takes place, the kneecap points towards the outside of the body and the foot becomes more and more rigid as the arch is raised. External rotation takes place until lift-off, at which time internal rotation begins again.

Another event occurs which is of primary importance in walking and running. In the middle of the stance phase of gait, everything becomes neutral (*Figures 5 and 6*). Everything lines up ideally if the person has a neutral foot structure (very few runners have) and everything is balanced (*Figure 7*). In most people this balancing act does not take place on time or to the full extent that it should. This causes the imbalance and overuse syndromes which we will talk about throughout the book.

As the runner proceeds from walking to jogging and to faster running, the amount of time the stance-phase foot is on the ground decreases and an airborne phase becomes more evident (*Figure 8*). A jogger usually has a "heel-foot-toe" cadence or may have a "foot-toe" type of gait. Faster runners spend most of their time on the balls of their feet. A middle-distance runner

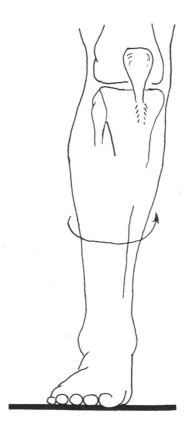

FIGURE 4
Prolonged Pronation of the Foot

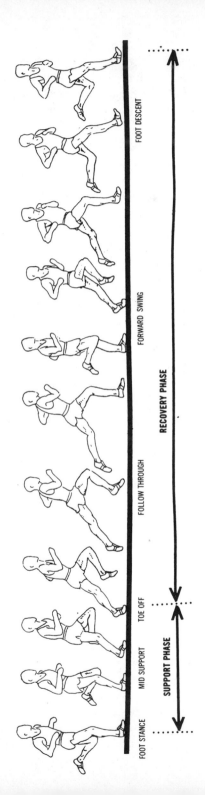

FIGURE 5

The Gait Cycle in Running

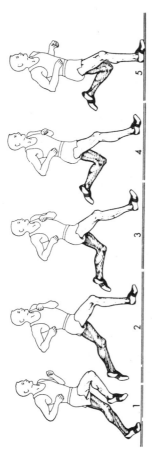
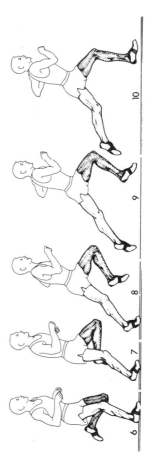

FIGURE 6
Biomechanics of Running

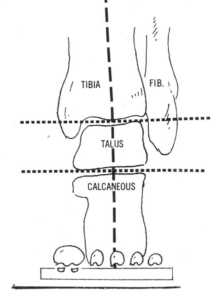

FIGURE 7

The Normal Foot and Leg

may contact on the ball of the foot, rock back on the heel, then have a powerful lift-off.

A biomechanical approach allows walkers and runners without normal foot-leg structure to contact on the outside of the heel (anywhere from 1-3 degrees), to roll in (pronate) to help absorb shock and allow the foot to be a mobile adapter, then to externally rotate the leg again and allow the foot to become a more rigid lever for a normal lift-off. All of this is accomplished by making some form of a device to bring the surface up to meet what we consider to be a functionally neutral foot.

This means the position that the foot should be held in, for best function of every individual runner, must be found and must be held by some form of foot support or foot orthotic. This allows for the bony structures and joints as well as ligaments and muscles of the lower extremity to provide for their own stability.

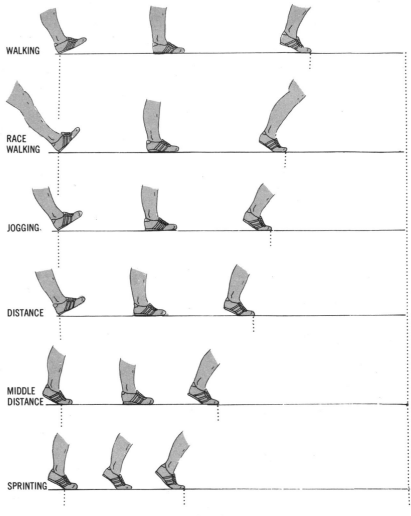

FIGURE 8

Comparison of Walking, Jogging, Sprinting

6

Feet I Meet

Every foot is different. Every foot has its own characteristics, its own print, arch and flexibility. Every foot has its own function and its own characteristic biomechanical properties. Every foot functions just a bit different from every other.

But feet can be grouped into broad categories, just as every other subject in science. These help us explain things better. Basic categories have a tendency to respond similarly to basic stresses and basic treatments for these stresses. Not all, but many feet have functions and types which can be generalized. These may help us to understand the biomechanics of injury and sports medicine.

NEUTRAL FOOT

The neutral foot is the ideal foot. "Neutral" means that the foot has intrinsic stability due to its position when both feet are on the ground. (We call this "bipedal stance.") When the heel is perpendicular to the ground and the arch is normal and the metatarsal heads rest on the ground, the arch stability is maintained by the neutral position of the bones in the foot. Intrinsic, inborn stability maintained by neutral joints means that the muscles do not have to support the arch or support body weight.

It appears, then, that a neutral arch and foot is less likely to have overuse injuries associated with its function because the muscles don't have to work overtime or become overused.

Obviously, motion precludes bipedal stance. If you are to

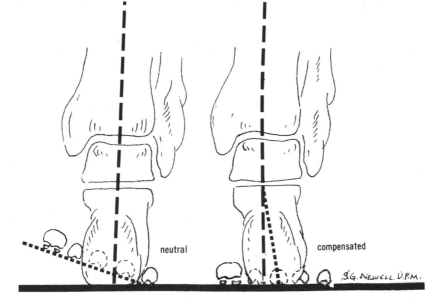

FIGURE 1

Forefoot Varus and Compensation

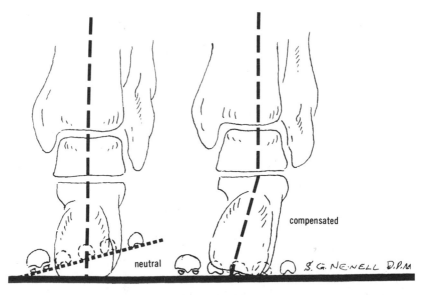

FIGURE 2

Forefoot Valgus and Compensation

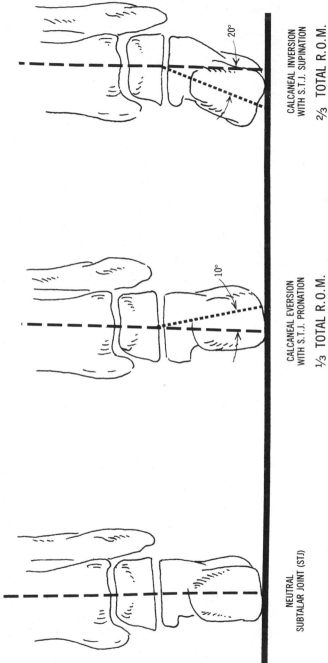

NEUTRAL
SUBTALAR JOINT (STJ)

CALCANEAL EVERSION
WITH S.T.J. PRONATION

1/3 TOTAL R.O.M.

CALCANEAL INVERSION
WITH S.T.J. SUPINATION

2/3 TOTAL R.O.M.

10°

20°

FIGURE 3

Neutral Position of Subtalar Joint

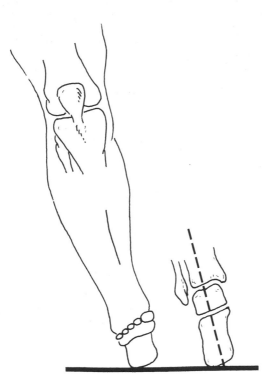

FIGURE 4

Tibial Varum

move, one foot has to be doing just the opposite of the other foot. Both feet cannot be neutral as the same time during walking, jogging or running. The foot, during motion, is neutral only at the middle of the time the foot is on the ground. However, for everything to work in sequence, for motion to be orderly and function around the neutral base line, the foot must be neutral at the correct time. Otherwise, the overuse and imbalance injuries may occur.

IRREGULARITIES

All feet have a neutral position. Most of these neutral positions place the foot tilted from the ground. In other words, the foot is neutral, but some portions of the foot are not in full contact with the ground.

An example of this is what we call "forefoot varus," in which

---

the first, second and maybe third metatarsal heads do not contact the weight-supporting surface when the remainder of the foot is neutral (*Figures 1, 2, 3 and 4*).

Thus, we build a foot orthotic or support device to bring the ground to the foot. This orthotic foot device allows the foot to have its own stability. This is an interesting concept which should be understood, since it is the key to preventing overuse injuries. The foot becomes stable through proper joint positioning.

Podiatrists type feet by how they line up when they are neutral. Patients are examined while lying on their stomachs to see how the neutral joint positions line up with each other, and then they are examined when walking, running and standing to see how the neutral joint positions line up to the floor. This is used also to see the difference between how they are functioning and how they *should* function in a more neutral position.

In the case studies to come, we'll look at the many things that go wrong because of improper function, and what can be done about them.

7

The Forefoot

Forefoot biomechanics or balance can be discussed through two basic foot types—the rigid forefoot or flexible forefoot.

Flexible forefoot. It may be so flexible that it results in excessive pronation during movement, with pronatory overuse syndromes being the result. Dr. Dudley Morton, and more recently Dr. George Sheehan, refer to this as the "atavistic" or "Morton's" foot. I prefer to define the extent of the problem by the angle that the metatarsal heads make with the floor and heel when the foot is "neutral." This is called "forefoot varus." These angles are most useful when considering foot orthotic design and function.

Trends suggest that a forefoot varus of 6-7 degrees causes the runner to be restless when standing still and more comfortable when pacing or moving, yet even more at home when walking on uneven surfaces. I have forefoot varus, and before I made my first pair of orthotics in 1967 I couldn't stand still for more than 30 minutes. My legs would ache during longer surgeries, the backs of my legs would knot up, the tight bands of tissue ached beneath the skin on the soles of my feet. My foot posture was at fault.

Why? Forefoot varus means that there is an angle between the ground and the inside metatarsal heads when the foot is neutral. With all the body weight going through the foot during stance, and even more weight during running (4-6 times the body weight), it becomes apparent that the metatarsal heads will have to touch the floor. In fact, they will be *forced* to the floor. This causes strain to the arch as well as the leg, which must rotate inward more than normal as the arch lowers.

Foot orthotics bring the ground to the forefoot, stabilize the foot, and the strain is gone. In my case, the change was dramatic. I can stand for prolonged periods without fatigue (though I still enjoy pacing). If I don't wear my orthotics, after an hour or so I begin feeling foot and leg fatigue.

Forefoot varus usually produces a noticeable foot complaint, such as arch strain, heel spur syndrome or bunions, along with leg complaints of runner's knee and inside leg (posterior tibial and flexor) shin splint syndrome. Forefoot varus-related stress fractures in the metatarsals and lower leg also are common.

The ideal foot has no forefoot varus, but the average person has 3-4 degrees. In this amount, it responds well to orthotics. However, forefoot varus of 10 degrees or more becomes much harder to treat, and runners with this much deformity have had few pain-free moments. Something in the foot or leg has always hurt. The achilles tendon is usually secondarily tight and frequently strained. The ankle hurts on the insides.

Ten degrees is enough deformity so that limits of correction which can be tolerated by the feet are reached. I have had to compromise in these cases and construct semi-pronated orthotics, usually with a heel lift, to help these runners. Their feet are not neutral in the orthotics, but they are not as pronated as before the orthotics. There is a position between neutral and pronated which takes care of most of the running overuse symptoms, and the podiatrist has the job of finding this functional bio-mechanics position.

Rigid forefoot. This causes "forefoot valgus," which is the opposite of the forefoot varus in appearance and in cause. The outside metatarsal heads fail to touch the ground. The foot compensates by "supinating" (the opposition of pronating), the arch becomes higher and more rigid and the leg must externally rotate. The plantar fascia (tight bands beneath the skin of the arch) may tear or rupture. Calluses form beneath rigid metatarsal heads. The big toe joint may jam with limited motion. The ankle sprains more easily, and the outside of the legs, knee and hip may be more prone to strain. This foot absorbs strain poorly. Therefore, shock is transmitted to the upper leg and thigh.

This foot may do well with a rigid orthotic for walking but may need a more flexible support for running, especially if the plantar fascia is tight. The support stabilizes the outside border of the foot and reduces the over-supination. This allows the foot to be more flexible.

Too much rigidity as well as too much flexibility are weak links in the running cycle. A foot must be flexible at heel contact, yet rigid at lift-off to function well. The foot is constantly changing between these two extremes during function. When imbalance is present, foot orthotics allow the foot to make those normal and essential functional changes.

8

The Rearfoot

There are various types of orthotic control: (1) *forefoot control,* which takes care of forefoot valgus and forefoot varus; (2) *arch control,* which keeps the arch from collapsing, and (3) *rearfoot control,* which regulates the rolling in and rolling out or "pitch" of the heel bone.

Various types of materials can be used to achieve control. I may use a bulky material such as felt to push up the arch, and I may secure it with tape. Likewise, the tape may be used fairly effectively to help give some form of rearfoot control.

However, the most effective type of control is accomplished with a "rearfoot post" on an orthotic. A post is a balancing device, usually made of plastic or rubber. It works best when it is molded onto a rigid plastic support, though orthotics of this type don't adapt well to all sports. I have found, for instance, that a plastic support is quite adequate for slow distance running and everyday use. However, faster running and jumping may require softer orthotics in which the heel-controlling properties are compromised.

It is necessary with rigid orthotics to know the warning signs of too much or too little rearfoot control. Ideally, a rearfoot post allows the runner to contact on the outside of the heel anywhere from 2-4 degrees supinated, and then to roll in to 2-4 degrees of pronation. Total motion is normally 6-8 degrees. The orthotics must allow this much motion, neither more nor less. Overuse injuries occur from errors in either direction.

There is a position around which every foot functions best. If the foot isn't already in that position, it may require rearfoot control. The podiatrist must decide the best functional position of the calcaneus (heel bone), and then support it in that position.

I had a patient, a runner for an Ivy League school, who came to me with ailments resulting from congenital flat feet. He also had an inborn tightness of the achilles tendons, and he could not stretch out the tendons with exercise. He complained of agonizing pulling and repeated strains of the posterior tibial muscles. As he ran, his heel cords were so tight, they forced the foot to become even more pronated, which caused the pulling of the tibial muscles.

I casted his foot in the pronated position. This isn't normal procedure, but in his case I could not put him in the neutral position because his "neutral" would have placed abnormal stress on the achilles tendon. He either would have ended up breaking down his orthotics or forming ulcers at the arches where the orthotics were pushing up. His achilles tendons probably would have become even more symptomatic.

In this case, the rearfoot post held his heel pronated about four degrees. I also raised the heel with a heel lift. This worked well. The runner returned to his college team and ran better than before he had worn orthotics.

The big mistake I see being made with rigid orthotics is too much control. It is far better to have too little control and too much pronation than to err in the other direction. Too much control limits contact pronation, which is necessary to dissipate stress. The mechanism for unlocking the joints (thereby dispersing contact force) must be left intact. This mechanism relies upon a good six degrees of contact pronation.

With too much rearfoot control, there is excessive tilting of the calcaneus to the outside. Contact pronation is limited, and shock waves are transmitted throughout the foot, leg, knee and thigh. These may lead to overuse syndromes in places a runner has never had them before. A key warning sign of overcontrol is a strain at the outside of the knee. A strain also may appear at the outside of the hip.

What can be done if there appears to be too much control? Simply grind down the inside of the rearfoot post.

9

Finding Support

Some basic rules and concepts about orthotics should be understood. The most important one is this foot support is not a crutch. Actually, "foot support" is a misnomer, because the orthotic does not support the foot; it merely allows the foot to get into the proper positions so that the muscles can do their job in aligning the joints, and the bony architecture of the foot can do its job in actually supporting the body weight.

This is why we use the term "functional orthotics." They cause the foot to function better. There is no actual muscle or arch weakening as a result of wearing a foot orthotic. In fact, because there is better phasic activity and muscle function, the lower extremities become stronger.

The next important factor is that as the rigidity and sophistication of the foot orthotic increases, so does the biomechanical control. Those who have a high degree of foot deformity will have dramatic relief of their overuse syndromes with almost any type of support. But as the foot approaches the norm, it becomes more difficult to control it with anything but a rather sophisticated functional orthotic. This, by definition, must be of a more rigid material.

What problems do we have with rigid foot orthotics? One of the more common is that they squeak. This is especially true of the plastic supports. The squeaking is caused by friction between the shoe and the support, and is handled in almost all cases simply by applying some type of foot or body powder between the orthotic and the shoe. (I like to put powder on the top of the orthotic, too.)

Sometimes, the orthotics appear to be too wide for the shoe. Actually, the shoe is too narrow for the foot, but most people won't accept this fact. We have found it necessary to alter the orthotics at times to fit the various shoes on the market. I like to have an orthotic which can be used for everyday shoes and running so that one pair of orthotics are all that is necessary for an average runner for the rest of his life, provided it is made properly the first time around.

Some people find that their orthotics fit fine in their running shoes but will not fit in their everyday shoes. They fail to realize that their everyday shoes are probably too small to begin with and with a foot orthotic they should go up to a half a size to a full size. This may also hold true for their running shoes, since a size is somewhat less than one-quarter inch.

When the heel rides up and down in the shoe, we find it works well to remove the insole of the shoe underneath the rearfoot post. If there is a blistering problem or edge on the inside edge of the foot, the rubber arch pads in the shoe may be to blame and should be removed. When there is abnormal wear to the outside of the shoe heel, this might mean that there is too much control in the orthotic and it will need some form of adjustment.

When the top of the foot aches with a new orthotic, this is often from pressure of a tight-fitting shoe and a larger shoe will be necessary. When there is lateral strain at the knee joint, leg or hip, then the orthotic is giving too much control and not allowing enough contact pronation. A simple adjustment to allow pronation will take care of this problem.

The blister problem with orthotics appears to be handled fairly well by applying synthetic materials such as Spenco which absorb stress. Bony prominences may have to be accommodated for by heating the orthotic and pressing the plastic away from these prominences.

Patients who have tight heel cords and compensate for them by pronating their foot may find even more discomfort in the heel cords with their new orthotics, unless they do proper stretching exercises. Those people who have congenitally short heel cords, however, will not tolerate a neutral foot support and must have pronated support. At times, they must even have an additional heel lift.

It is important to realize that when you get into an orthotic, your angle of gait is going to change. You will most likely be more pigeon-toed or in-toed. This causes the limbs to rotate differently. At first, there may be a mild amount of hip pain or low back pain associated with the new orthotics. Usually, proper exercising will take care of this problem.

What exactly do the orthotics do? The orthotics appear to work extremely well for overuse syndromes of the leg, knee, thigh, hip and back. They also work wonders on the foot in regards to heel spur syndrome and functional tarsal tunnel. They usually help plantar fasciitis, but there may be times when they aggravate the plantar fascia. I have had instances in which a runner switches from slow distance training to intervals, and uses his plastic orthotics. The plastic may actually cause irritation to the fascia, which tightens as the runner gets up on the balls of his feet. For speed training, I generally recommend a semi-flexible or soft orthotic.

I am of the opinion that almost every athlete could benefit from some form of foot support or some form of shock-absorbing material within the shoes. It actually startles me when I read the statement, because it appears to oversell something I do—that is, taking care of biomechanical problems and at times utilizing various materials to control lower extremity function. But, athletes should have the best protection available when their health and performance are at stake.

part III

THE INJURY LIST

10

Skin and Nails

BLISTERS

Despite their lowly status, the most common foot problem in runners is blisters. I have seen blisters completely cripple runners.

Continuous friction causes separation of the layers of skin or actual sheering between the outer layer of the skin (epidermis) and the lower layer (dermis). The warning sign of blisters is redness or a "hot spot" on the foot, and the runner usually knows when he is going to get one.

"Breaking in" orthotics may cause blisters. We find this with soft orthotics as well as with the plastic orthotics. When a patient has soft orthotics and is getting a blister, we simply check to see how the orthotics are fitting in the shoes. Often, we find that the runner has failed to take the sponge rubber padding from the running shoes, and this is causing an additional lift on the arch of the soft orthotic. Simply removing the soft rubber will take care of the problem. Rigid orthotics generally are covered with Spenco material when they are dispensed in my office. This normally prevents any blister formation. Spenco insoles help eliminate blistering in those who don't wear orthotics as well.

Vaseline also might help. I recall running the Boston Marathon in 1976, when it was so hot that the spectators hosed off the runners. This caused my shoes and socks to become very wet. The wet socks caused quite a bit of blistering before the end of the race. Dr. John Pagliano, a sports podiatrist from Long Beach, Calif., suggested that half a handful of Vaseline rubbed on each foot prior to running would help. He said a pair of medium-thickness cotton socks allow the Vaseline to ooze through and form a friction barrier between the foot and the shoe.

Treatment of blisters depends upon the location. If they are on the toes and not bothersome, I suggest that they should be left alone and not popped. If they are painful, with fluid accumulating in them, they can be cleansed with Phisohex and water or alcohol and lanced, with the skin not being removed, then again cleansed. I prefer using tape on these if you're going for a run. Likewise, painful blisters on the bottom of the feet with fluid should be lanced, decompressed, cleansed with soap and water, and then covered with moleskin, tape or gauze with tape over it.

CALLUSES

Another skin problem is calluses, which usually are caused by abnormal movement of the metatarsal heads. There are two types of calluses, the "friction callus" and the "sheering callus." Calluses are always the result of a biomechanical problem if they are under bony prominences, especially beneath the metatarsal heads. Calluses on the heels usually are carried by improper gait patterns. Calluses can be treated well with orthotics though at times surgical procedures are necessary to remove severe calluses to underlying bony prominences.

NAILS

Nail problems are more disfiguring than disabling. The hallmark of many runners is their black toenails or toenails which are falling off. Runners who use hills may get black nails as their feet slide forward in the shoes while going downhill. Runners who buy their shoes too tight may have trauma to the toenails with subsequent bleeding beneath the toenails, which gives the black color. One painful condition of the toenails is the "subungual hematoma" or the blood clot beneath the nail. This usually has to be drained and may be done simply by heating a paperclip and pushing the clip through the nail. The blood spurts out through the nail, relieving the pressure that had caused pain. Soaking the nail after this will usually take care of the problem.

Sometimes, runners get ingrown toenails on the great toes secondary from shoes which are too narrow in the toe area. The chronic rubbing of the soft tissue on the nail causes the nail to dig into the skin, and a secondary infection occurs. The nail then becomes a foreign body and must be partially removed in the area of ingrowing. If ingrowing continues, then the matrix or cells from which the nail grows can be removed in one area, leaving a normal-appearing nail which does not grow in. Your podiatrist can help you with these problems.

FOOT ODOR

Runners also may have problems with their feet sweating too much. We call this "hyperhydrosis." When the sweating is accompanied by a foul-smelling condition of the feet, we call this "bromhydrosis." I usually treat these problems with foot powder, two or three times a day, sprinkled inside of stockings. I have my patients wear moccasins or slippers around the house, with a liberal amount of foot powder applied to them. When the condition is quite severe, we utilize a 5% solution of formaldehyde applied at night with cotton swabs. It completely dries out the feet. A commercial medication called "Dry Sol" can be applied at night, once a week to feet which are then covered with Saran Wrap. This works extremely well.

OTHER COMPLAINTS

Occasionally, runners have athlete's foot, which is a fungal infection. This is best treated by prescription medications for the fungus as well as over-the-counter athlete's foot or fungal powder. It often is necessary to take a culture of the fungus to identify the exact nature of the infection so that proper treatment can be instituted.

Warts are a common skin problem and usually are removed with acid solutions by a podiatrist.

EVAN GOLDER CASE

Evan Golder works as a minister and a writer. He was never an athlete in his younger years and did not start running until he was 30 years old, when he found himself in a sedentary job. He joined a physical fitness program at the YMCA and began jogging around the gym. When the gym became too small for him, he ran around the block. When the block became too small, he ran around Lake Merritt. When the lake became too small, he took to the open road. Since then, he has run 10 marathons.

Evan first came to my office in March 1975, complaining of pain on the bottom of his left foot. This pain felt like a pebble in his shoe when he ran. He was running 5-10 miles daily, and the pain had been present for six weeks.

My examination revealed that he had a wart ("plantar ver-rucae") beneath the fourth metatarsal head of his left foot. Apparently, the metatarsal head had been rubbing the bottom of his foot in the shoe and the skin broke down, allowing a virus to cause a wart. The reason I could recognize a wart rather than a callus was that, when I trimmed it down, there was a lot of pinpoint bleeding. The wart hurt more with lateral pinching than with direct pressure. This is characteristic.

Treatment consisted of blocking the foot with Xylocaine and removing the wart with blunt dissection, with care being taken not to form any scar tissue. Evan was given soft orthotics to pad around the metatarsal heads and to help build up the arches of the feet.

The wart healed completely, and upon reviewing Evan's x-rays and noting his feet when he walked, I suggested he might do well with a pair of plastic orthotics to possibly prevent any further running injuries. But he was so comfortable in the soft orthotics that he thought he would stay with them for a while.

Evan returned to my office more than a year later. He said the soft orthotics didn't make him feel that much better but that he felt bad when not wearing them. This is an interesting way to describe what the orthotics are doing. He also suggested that, when running marathons, he lost one or two toenails prior to getting the orthotics but that with the orthotics his feet moved less in his shoes and he had not lost a nail. He wanted to be casted for the rigid orthotics. Not everybody takes this much time to realize he needs a more permanent type of control, but it is always best, in my opinion, to let the patient decide on what he wants in regard to orthotics. I just give suggestions.

11

Big-Toe Bunions

JAMES HENRY

James Henry was a 64-year-old who had only one desire in life when he first came to see me. That was to run the Dipsea Race. He had the ability and the strength. There was only one thing holding him back, his bunions (*Figure 1*). His great toes did not articulate well with the rest of his foot. He had so much stiffness, in fact, that it was getting very difficult for him to run. His mileage had been cut down from six miles a day, to three, to one, and finally to just a half-mile. He just didn't have enough flexibility in these joints to allow proper running.

James had arthritis secondary to overuse and biomechanical deformity, which is known as "hallux limitus." There was a sandpaper-type feeling when moving the big toe up and down, motion was quite limited, and painful. X-rays of his feet showed that the joints were quite narrow and that there was arthritis in both great toe joints. I discussed this problem with him at length, and we both decided it would be best to operate on the feet and actually build him joints.

The surgery required remodeling the first metatarsal phalangeal joint and forming a new joint by placing a medical-grade plastic joint or "spacer" in the great toes. Along with this, it was necessary to form new grooves on the bottom of the first metatarsal heads for the small sesamoid bones which are necessary to provide for power and spring.

This surgery was carried out in 1973. James recently told me that he'd had no problems with his feet in three years. He was running as fast as he pleased, and was very happy with the surgery—the first case where implants were used on an athlete.

BEN HIRSCH

Ben Hirsch found new life when he became a distance runner after retirement. Now in his mid-70s, he runs from 25-40 miles per week, has run several marathons and has raced up Pike's Peak.

Ben came to my office in October 1973, complaining of abnormal heel wear on his running shoes as well as sharp pain from the right back down to the right foot. He'd had this for two or three months. He also had bunions which were somewhat painful in the wrong shoes.

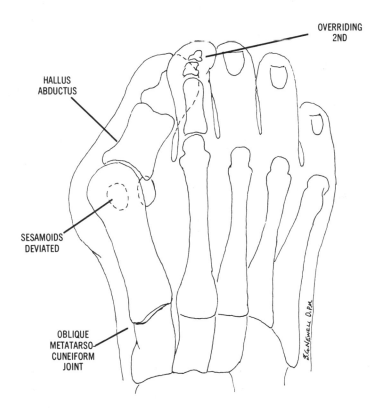

OVERRIDING 2ND

HALLUS ABDUCTUS

SESAMOIDS DEVIATED

OBLIQUE METATARSO-CUNEIFORM JOINT

FIGURE 1

Hallus Valgus with Bunion

My examination revealed that Ben's bunions were somewhat inflamed and grossly deformed. His second toes lay on top of his great toes. We call this a "hallux valgus" with overlapping second toes (*Figure 1*). This basically means that the great toes are bent toward the outside of the feet and the second toes lie on top of them. The bunion is the protrusion of bone on the inside of the foot at the big toe joint. Pressure from the shoe causes this to be red, inflamed and tender.

In Ben's case, this was so bad that the joint also had some arthritis in it. Due to the bunion and the instability of the great toe, there was a callus underneath the second metatarsal head. This is a type of Morton's foot. He had a moderate amount of instability of both feet.

Further examination revealed that the left leg was five-eighths inch shorter than the right. This might have been contributing to the sciatic-type nerve pain on the right side. When he walked, his feet were turned outward about 15 degrees. This is not unusual for people who are over the age of 40, since they need more stability if they have not been active and gain this by rolling their feet to the outside.

We made soft orthotics for him. I also built special pads to protect his bunions and his second toes. He was given a heel lift for the short right leg. It appeared to me that a 71-year-old man as active as Ben might do better with having his shoes adjusted rather than his feet adjusted. In other words, I preferred not to do surgery if it could at all have been avoided.

Ben came back several months later, noting that he was doing quite well with the supports but that his second toe was digging into the great toe due to the deformity. I readjusted the bunion pads and these appeared to work quite well. When he returned in July 1974, he was complaining of bunion pain due to the pressure of the shoes, but he still was running from 4-8 miles. At this time, I made special bunion shields of rubber from a cast of the foot. These worked well.

The lesson to be learned here: There are various conservative measures which can be carried out to make somebody remain active and comfortable rather than resorting to surgery. Surgery is sometimes necessary, but conservative, non-surgical treatment should be exhausted before resorting to surgical procedures.

BETSY WHITE

Betsy White had been running for three years and had run marathons when she came to see me in 1975. She complained of a painful left bunion and, in addition, wanted to have a preventive checkup and possible treatment to waylay any future injuries.

When I first saw Betsy, her bunion wasn't causing a grating sensation which we call "crepitation." When crepitation is present, the prognosis is not so good since there is arthritis in the joint. Betsy did not appear to have arthritis, but rather an inflammation of the tissue on the side of the foot, secondary to what appeared to be a malposition of the great toe. The bunion deformity was worse when she was standing with her foot pronated than when we realigned her foot with a normal arch. It was apparent, then, that some form of arch control might prevent her bunion from getting worse.

Biomechanically, Betsy had about two degrees of instability in the rearfeet and seven degrees of forefoot varus. This is a rather excessive amount of forefoot varus and needs orthotics for control.

Treatment consisted of placing Betsy in a functional plastic orthotic to control the forefoot varus and Morton's foot syndrome. The results were quite good, as the bunion pain disappeared. I saw Betsy at the Boston Marathon in 1976, where I just happened to pass her with about a hundred yards left in the race.

It is important to realize that pain in the feet is a warning sign that something is wrong. The bunion pain means that something is definitely in need of treatment. In Betsy's case, we were lucky. It appears that we prevented bunion surgery.

12

Nerve Damage

PAULETTE SHARP

Paulette Sharp, a 28-year-old nursing student, came to my office in May 1975 complaining of pain in both feet, more so on the right foot. The pain appeared to be centered at the bottom of her foot, in the space where the third and fourth toes meet the rest of the forefoot.

She had noted that the pain first occurred while she ran on the beach a few days before the Bay-to-Breakers race. She ran the race and could barely walk afterwards. For the past two weeks, she had been recuperating and in the past two or three days had started running again with dull aching in the right foot.

My examination of the right foot revealed tenderness and pain with the pressure of my fingers in the third interspace under the ball of the foot. I felt a clicking mass. As I moved this mass, Paulette experienced pain which shot into her toes. The left foot had a similar feeling but less pain.

Biomechanically, her feet had 5-6 degrees of forefoot varus, which is a moderate amount, and she pronated somewhat excessively. Otherwise, her feet were fairly normal. She had good flexibility.

My diagnosis was that of Morton's interdigital neuroma (*Figure 1*), on both feet, more severe on the right. I also wanted to make sure she did not have a stress fracture or some bone problem which can present similar symptoms. But x-rays showed no bone problems whatsoever.

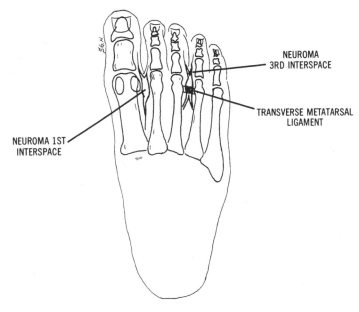

FIGURE 1

Interdigital Neuroma

I prescribed soft, temporary, flexible orthotics to see whether supports would help her condition. If these didn't work, we would perform cortisone injections into the interspaces to soften scar tissue around the nerve. Paulette returned the next week and said the soft orthotics had been causing some blistering problems, but that her feet felt much better. The soft orthotics were adjusted and she was told to return to the office if she decided to have more rigid orthotics.

We received a photo from Paulette recently, showing her running in a race. She had not come back to the office, so apparently she had done well in the soft supports. The soft supports eventually will wear down and she may need a new pair of soft orthotics or may need to be casted for the rigid orthotics which will last longer and provide better control. But her problem was caught early enough that conservative treatment was successful.

If there had been extensive damage to the nerves or a great deal of scar tissue, they would have been removed surgically. In such cases, runners usually return to running in 2-3 weeks.

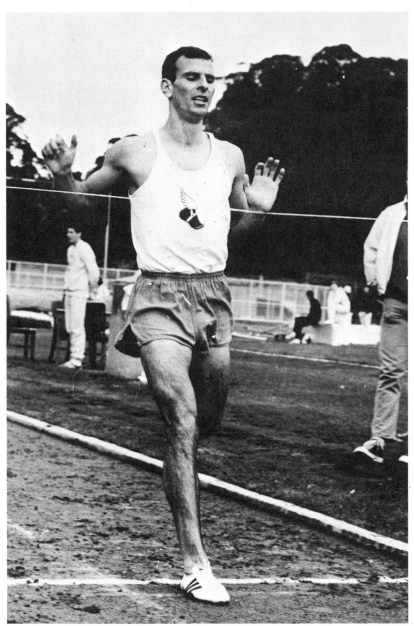

Tom Laris, Olympian in 1968 and later a professional, was slowed in recent years by neuromas.

Jeff Kroot

BILL CLARK

Bill Clark has been a world class runner, second in the Boston Marathon, an American record-holder in several events. I was very impressed at having such a good runner in my office.

Bill complained of a right foot pain in the second interspace, and on both feet painful third toes. He noticed most of his pain was at toe-off in running. It had become worse in recent months, and this was affecting his high-mileage training.

Examination of his feet showed a Morton's neuroma present in the second interspace of the right foot and in both third interspaces. There were clicking masses in these interspaces; these were painful to the touch. These neuromas actually were inflammations surrounding the normal nerves of the foot, which resulted from increased mileage and pressure on the nerves when running on the ball of the foot. X-rays of the feet showed no bone pathology, other than Morton's feet with lowering of the arch. X-rays also showed hypermobility of the first metatarsal, which goes along with the Morton's foot syndrome.

Bill was placed in soft orthotics. When he returned two weeks later, the neuromas still hurt, so I used a mixed cortisone injection in the interspaces to decrease the inflammation around the nerves.

On his next visit, the neuromas were better, but still hurt. I gave him injections again, and at that time he began using plastic orthotics. The next time I saw him, the neuromas were much better. They still could be felt but appeared to be disappearing. The orthotics were adjusted.

By April, four months after his first visit, the neuromas were no longer painful. His neuromas have been asymptomatic since then. He had been using plastic orthotics, mostly for walking, and the softer orthotics for fast running. Bill races at around a five-minute pace, and he noted that for his type of running, on the balls of the feet, he needed a flexible orthotic.

TOM LARIS

Tom Laris is a pro. He ran on the professional track circuit and has been a member of the United States Olympic team in the 10,000-meter run. Tom was 35 years old when he first visited my office in October 1975. He had pain between the toes on the bottom of the foot, at the second interspace, right side. He had

---

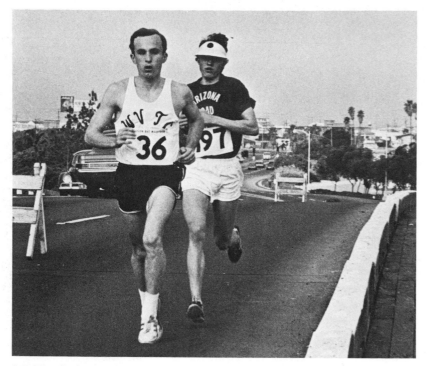

Bill Clark (left) suffered from a number of foot and leg ailments after setting American records in the early 1970s.

been running only 55 miles per week (low for him), but doing a lot of speed work up on the balls of his feet. The pain was so severe that he could not run much more than six miles, whereas two months earlier he could run 15 miles without pain in the foot.

My examination revealed a clicking mass in the painful area, suggesting a Morton's interdigital neuroma or inflammation around the nerve. X-rays were taken which showed no real bone pathology, only Morton's foot. Biomechanical examination showed moderate flattening of the feet with six degrees forefoot varus and 2-3 degrees rearfoot varus. Tom had the problem of being bow-legged, with seven degrees tibial varum.

Treatment consisted of a mixed cortisone (long-acting and short-acting) injection around the nerve to soften the scar tissue, and soft orthotics for speedwork and rigid orthotics for everyday use. He needed a series of three weekly spaced injections which he disliked greatly but which helped his condition.

I explained to Tom that if he wanted to increase his mileage he probably would need to have this neuroma removed. He decided against it but got well enough so he could run up to 15 miles without pain.

When I talked with Tom recently, he informed me that his feet are totally asymptomatic. My conclusion from this is that the nerve irritation he was having must have been due to abnormal pronation of the foot, with secondary irritation to the nerves. Apparently, the orthotics straightened out this problem.

13

Forefoot Pain

DOMINGO TIBADUIZA

Domingo Tibaduiza came to my office about two weeks after the 1976 Olympics with a very painful left foot. The Colombian Olympian complained of pain in the region of the second metatarsal phalangeal joint (where the second toe meets the foot). He noted that the toe was somewhat bent and appeared to be pushed over towards the side, closer to the great toe.

About two months earler, he'd noticed pain in the foot which gradually had become worse until it had affected his training and ultimately his performance at Montreal.

There was no specific pain or redness along the bone itself. Had there been, this might have suggested a stress fracture which should have been healed after two months. There was, however, some pain over the tendons on the top of the foot to the second toe. This suggested an extensor tendonitis. Likewise, there was swelling around the joint. This suggested some form of arthritis or "capsulitis" (inflammation of the capsule covering the joint). There was pain to each side of the second metatarsal head and some clicking sensations, which could have been neuromas in the first and second interspaces. Perhaps the most significant finding was a rather large, thick callus under the second and third metatarsal heads on the left foot.

Domingo had a moderate amount of imbalance in his feet, with a Morton's foot configuration which was worse on the left foot.

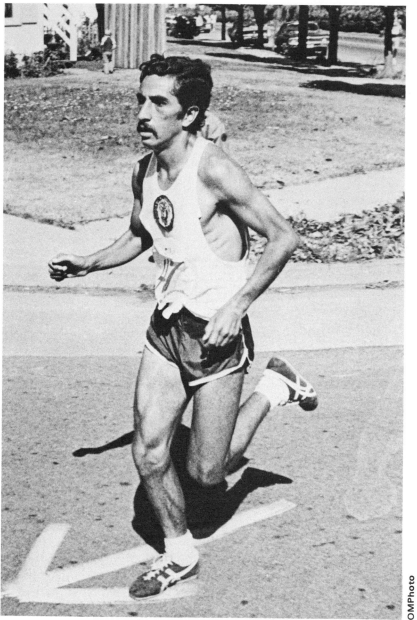

Domingo Tibaduiza, a Colombian Olympian, worried that his foot problem would hamper him for the rest of his life.

He also appeared to have a bit shorter left leg and tended to roll it to the outside when running, as if stepping into a hole.

No stress fracture or healed stress fracture was seen on the x-rays. However, the Morton's foot was confirmed. Domingo had been given a soft temporary foot support extending from the heel to underneath the metatarsal heads and was told to try running. He noticed that running was more comfortable with the supports, but a mild amount of pain still was present.

We then injected mixed cortisone into the areas where suspected neuromas were and into the joint area for the capsulitis. Domingo was instructed to do only long, slow distance running for the next two weeks, at which time he would return for a more rigid type of orthotic to be used for distance training and everyday use. He would use the soft orthotics for speedwork and races.

Domingo was wondering if this foot problem was going to hamper him for the rest of his life. I told him that since the problem appeared to be caused by external rotation of the left foot, and a smaller amount of rotation in the right, proper bio-mechanical control should allow him to return to pain-free running.

Thinking about Domingo and the athletes in Olympics, it is apparent to me that selection of sports medicine doctors for the Olympic Team is more political than functional. In 1976, no podiatrist was officially chosen to go to the Olympics and help the United States Team or members of other teams, yet the majority of injuries were leg and foot injuries. This, of course, is the province of podiatry.

JANE FREDERICK

Jane Frederick is the U.S. record-holder in the pentathlon, and placed sixth in the 1976 Olympic Games. Several years ago, she was referred to me by a Colorado doctor. She complained of a great deal of pain at the inner edge of her left foot and ankle. She thought the pain was related to the achilles tendon. It radiated up and down the leg and foot from underneath the inside ankle bone and was aggravated by jumping. Of course, in the penta-thlon, jumping is rather important.

Jane's x-rays showed no real abnormal bony deformities, with the exception of mild to moderate pronation of the feet. Bio-mechanically, she had four degrees of rearfoot varus on the left, three degrees on the right and a forefoot valgus of 3-4 degrees on both feet. Ankle flexibility on the left foot was somewhat limited. I felt this was because she was guarding the whole left foot from the pain. She had six degrees of tibial varum, and had a tendency, when walking, to place a lot of stress on the outside of both heels.

New x-rays showed a possible old fracture of the joint beneath the ankle joint. There also was tenderness over the nerve which runs beneath the inner ankle bone and a tingling sensation when I tapped on the nerve with my fingers.

I came to the tentative diagnosis of a "tarsal tunnel syndrome (*Figure 1*), which is a compression of the nerves and vessels underneath the inner ankle bone, secondary to stress. Apparently, jumping and running had caused swelling of the tissues in

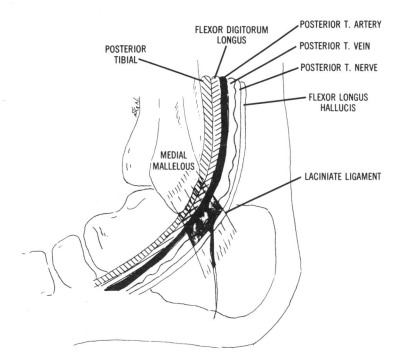

FIGURE 1

Tarsal Tunnel Syndrome

this area, which were pressing on the nerve and causing a radiating pain up and down the foot and leg.

I referred Jane to a neurologist for nerve conduction studies, to see if the nerve was performing properly. He said the conduction time was less on the left foot nerve than on the right, which suggested compression of the nerve.

Jane was casted, but the cast did not appear to make much difference. This made me think that what we assumed was a fracture was really an anatomical variation. Because of Jane's heavy competition schedule, she requested surgery if it would at all be helpful. She didn't want to wait through another season while we tried conservative measures.

At the time of surgery, I found that she did, indeed, have a very tight tarsal tunnel and that the nerve was being compressed. In addition, some of the tendons in that area

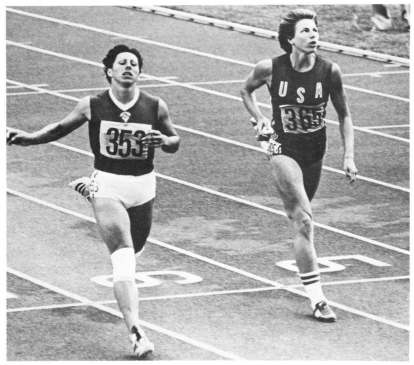

Mark Shearman

Jane Frederick (right) competed in the Olympics after foot surgery.

appeared to be inflamed and were in need of some surgical repair. Following the surgery in January 1973, she could again wiggle all toes without pain which hadn't been possible before.

After fitting Jane for new orthotics, I referred her back to her physician in Colorado. I have not heard from her again, but I assume the surgery must have been successful since she has been the leading American pentathlete since that time.

JEFFREY MILLER

Jeffry Miller, a skier and runner, came to me in August 1975, complaining of a large bump on the top of his left foot which hurt mostly when he wore ski boots. He also had pain over the fifth metatarsal head of the left foot. He noted that he had cracked a bone in 1969 while playing football and had pain off and on, at the top of his foot, since that time. He had not been treated for this problem.

My examination showed a large bump, which appeared to be a bone spur, at the point where the base of the first metatarsal hit the next bone, the first cuneiform. He also had enlargement of the outer edge of his fifth metatarsal head, and pressure from the shoes and boots was causing the skin to become red in this area. Eventually, he would have formed a callus in this area, because calluses are formed from pressures of this type.

X-rays confirmed the bony spurs which I saw in physical examination. Further examination showed that Jeff's first metatarsal was excessively mobile. During running, the pressure on the bottom of the metatarsal caused jamming at the top of the joint, which in turn led to more bone spur formation.

Although Jeff used orthotics he still had so much pain when wearing shoes that he required surgical removal of these spurs. The bump on the head of the fifth metatarsal also was removed.

When I saw him again several months later, he was doing extremely well with the exception of a small bump on his left foot. My examination showed that he had a cyst, which was quickly excised.

Jeff's case is interesting because it shows how previous trauma can cause bone spurs, which may need to be removed, and how simple excision of spurs gives good results.

14

Stress Fractures

HARRY CORDELLOS

Harry Cordellos is one of the country's more famous runners, inasmuch as he does not let his blindness limit him in any of his activities. Harry has a degree in physical education and can teach golf and diving. He is a long-distance runner who has broken the three-hour barrier in the marathon. He plays a guitar which he made himself. Harry obviously is a remarkable person and a pleasure to know.

I ran one race with Harry, over a very rough course. We also ran the race with elbows touching except over most difficult parts, where he actually grasped my elbow. The difficult parts included going down 45-degree slopes and at the same time jumping stumps and creeks. Harry didn't slow me down much. The only thing that slowed me down was my own lack of conditioning. During the whole race, which was approximately seven miles, Harry carried on a conversation and never once got out of breath.

I had known Harry for some time, but he first came to my office as a patient in May 1974. He had injured his left foot. He had noticed swelling and pain at the top of his left foot near the second and third metatarsal shafts.

Harry had run the Boston Marathon, then had come back two weeks later and run the Avenue of the Giants Marathon. His foot began hurting at 18 miles. He went ahead and finished, but his foot hurt so badly by then that he could barely walk.

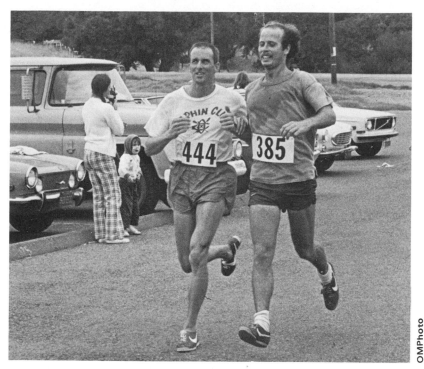

Foot troubles ended up interfering more with the running of Harry Cordellos (left) than his blindness did.

There now was redness and swelling over the top of the metatarsals, near the area where the metatarsal shaft meets the metatarsal head. Just by looking at his foot and hearing his history, I made a differential diagnosis of either a stress fracture of the second or third metatarsal or a tendonitis of the extensors, which are the tendons on the top of the foot. X-rays showed a very small crack, which I felt was a stress fracture. Such evidence is not extremely convincing, but the symptoms were bad enough that I suspected a stress fracture of the second metatarsal I treated him as though he had one.

I tried strapping the foot with tape, but when walking with this he still hurt. So I put him in a plaster of paris cast just around the foot itself. He wore this with a wooden shoe for two weeks and was able to ride a bike during this time. I then put him in a strapping which made him comfortable. I had him ride a bike for an additional week for resuming running.

Stress Fractures

Harry was getting quite nervous because the famous Bay-to-Breakers race was coming up and he didn't want to miss it. I made an accommodative pad out of felt, to put pressure on all the metatarsals except the second. I then strapped the foot with tape and told Harry he could start training for the race. About four days later, he ran the Bay-to-Breakers and had a great time. His foot did not hurt. He later returned to the office and got plastic orthotics which greatly have helped him in his running.

Biomechanically, Harry's motion is good, but he has a tendency to rotate his feet outward for stability. I suspect his blindness may have something to do with this. The plastic orthotics caused his feet to roll in, yet gave him enough stability where he ran faster and better. He has not been hurt since 1974.

It appears to me that the stress fracture might have occurred because Harry overdid it. Running a marathon, then coming back a week to two weeks later and running another marathon puts quite a bit of stress to the body. The constant microtrauma during running could have been enough to cause a crack in the bone. The fact that Harry ran through the marathon, even though he began hurting at 18 miles, further indicates that a small crack might have been converted into a larger crack and eventually a fracture.

RUTH ANDERSON

Ruth Anderson, who had always seemed indestructible, finally got hurt and came to me as a patient. She is one of the world's top over-40-year-old marathoners. In a race over extremely rugged terrain, she suffered an inversion injury with the foot turning under the leg. This resulted in a fracture of her fifth metatarsal.

Ruth was placed in a cast for one week. Then I removed the cast, strapped her foot and placed her in a semi-rigid support which was molded over the fracture site. The foot was held in a position of external rotation to minimize the pull of the muscle on the fracture site. X-rays showed that the fracture was in good alignment, and I assumed that if I could hold it there with a combination of strapping and the semi-rigid support, she would be able to use an exercise bike, do some walking and perhaps become more active.

Severe fractures take from 6-12 weeks to heal. However, I have

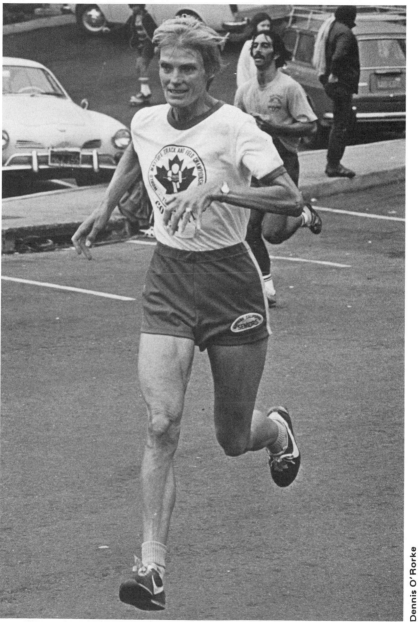

Marathoner Ruth Anderson, a world record-holder in her age group, fractured her foot during a mountain race.

Dennis O'Rorke

found that stress fractures or relatively non-involved fractures of the metatarsal bones in the foot may be knitted enough within three weeks to allow for some activity if a good foot support is provided as well as proper taping. In other words, we have let many of our runners jog on soft surfaces three weeks after a relatively benign fracture of a metatarsal.

This was my approach with Ruth. She was jogging three weeks after her injury. She returned to full-scale running very quickly, running in the national cross-country championships within two months of injury and the national marathon within three months.

15

Arch Injuries

PITTSBURGH EPISODE

In 1975 and '76, I ran the Boston Marathon. The American Medical Joggers Association had a three-day seminar on running medicine prior to each race, and the Road Runners of America also had its annual meeting in Boston. In 1975, I participated in the AMJA meeting, and in 1976 in both the AMJA and RRCA meetings.

My wife Jan and I have three children. Jan's parents live in Pittsburgh, so we left the children there and went on to Boston. In 1975, about one week prior to the Boston Marathon, I was running in Pittsburgh's Schenley Park. I noticed only one other runner on the rather hilly, coal-colored path—a tall, blonde young woman going in the opposite direction. I waved as we passed on the narrow trail.

The next year, at about the same time of the year, I again was running in Pittsburgh's Schenley Park. This time, I overtook the same woman and joined her for the last two miles of my eight-mile run. Her boyfriend was waiting at the finish with a stopwatch. He was a sub-three-hour marathoner who had not run for two months because of a foot injury. He had been injured in a marathon and had rested for two months following the onset of pain in his heels and inside arch where the fleshy muscle to the great toe attaches to the heel bone. After he learned I was a sports doctor, he said he must be treated immediately and run with me that day. Two months was too long to be off.

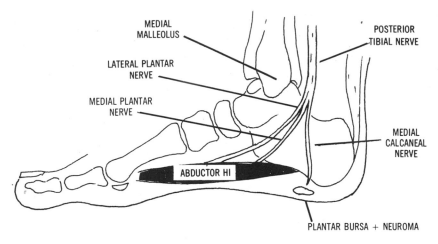

FIGURE 1

Heel Bruise and Arch Strain

I examined his foot on the lawn. Both feet had eight degrees of forefoot varus. The first metatarsals were hypermobile. The long toe was his second. He walked and ran with the heel bone pronated (everted) seven degrees. My impressions were that his heel bruise and arch strain were secondary to a weak Morton's foot (*Figure 1*).

We walked to the nearest drug store and purchased some Dr. Scholl's Flexo supports, moleskin, felt and tape. The store-bought supports didn't begin to support the arch until I added sufficient felt in the arch and inner heel (*Figure 2*). My friend had some bowleggedness with excessive outer heel wear in his shoes which to me suggested the need for an inner heel wedge or varus post (*Figure 3*). I used felt for these makeshift soft orthotics. The support helped greatly but not enough, so I used a tape arch strap (*Figure 4*) to rest the longitudinal arch.

All of this worked well, except that the heel was still a bit sore. The "stone bruise" was rather firm and organized with scar tissue. I injected a small amount of cortisone and Lidocaine into each heel, and we ran. My friend showed me old houses and cobblestone streets and stained-glass windows. It was a lovely day.

The next day, Jan and I flew to Boston.

GEORGE SHEEHAN

I'm on George Sheehan's mailing list. We became pen pals after meeting at a sports medicine seminar in San Francisco in 1973. We correspond regularly, and he sends me all of his columns from the *Red Bank (N.J.) Register.*

I had heard that somewhere in the East a cardiologist had been helped with his running injuries by podiatrist Richard Schuster. He now wished to convince the world that the foot is the "weak link" in most running injuries. I had to meet this Dr. Sheehan.

There, in the corner, somewhat withdrawn, the essence of the

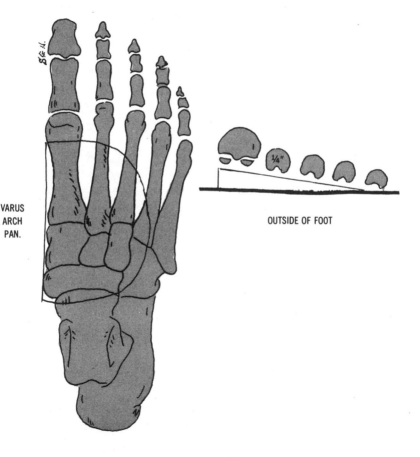

VARUS
ARCH
PAN.

OUTSIDE OF FOOT

Felt Arch Pad

ectomorphic long-distance runner, 10 pounds lighter than the insurance charts, stood George. Next to him was his wife, Mary Jane, mother of their 12 children.

So this was my hero. This was the man, complete with paper-clip as a tie tack. This was Podiatry's Friend. This was the author of the great book, *Encyclopedia of Sports Medicine.* We began talking, a dialogue that has never ended. The more George spoke, the more I listened. This *was* my hero.

Later that year, George came to the Bay Area and spent a week at my home. We ran two or three times a day and practiced medicine together at my office in Hayward. George read everything I had on podiatric sports medicine, we reviewed x-rays and

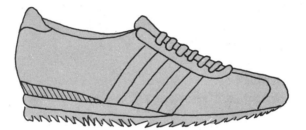

¼" FELT PAD

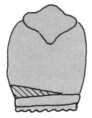

OUTSIDE OF HEEL

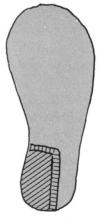

OUTSIDE OF HEEL

FIGURE 3

Quarter-Inch Felt Heel Pad

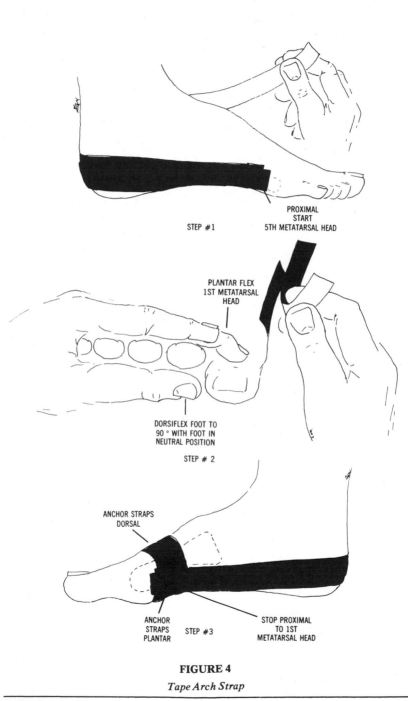

PROXIMAL
START
5TH METATARSAL HEAD

STEP #1

PLANTAR FLEX
1ST METATARSAL
HEAD

DORSIFLEX FOOT TO
90 ° WITH FOOT IN
NEUTRAL POSITION

STEP # 2

ANCHOR STRAPS
DORSAL

ANCHOR
STRAPS
PLANTAR

STEP #3

STOP PROXIMAL
TO 1ST
METATARSAL HEAD

FIGURE 4

Tape Arch Strap

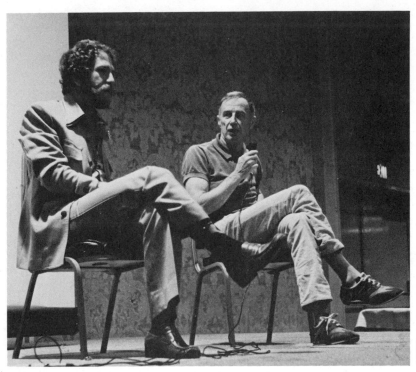

Dr. Subotnick (left) often shares the speaking platform with Dr. George Sheehan, "podiatry's friend."

slides, and I spoke to him of my interpretations of biomechanics and function. In return, he spoke to me of running philosophy, running medicine and the tasks that lay ahead of us to develop podiatry as a branch of sports medicine.

One day, George and I jogged over to the Cal State track and met Dennis Tracy for some 440 intervals. George ran hard. He likes to push himself. He gains insight from overcoming pain. He likes to run near the breaking point. After each 440, he would throw himself to the ground and pant while on all four limbs, chanting to God—presumably for forgiveness for the abuse he had given his body.

"Oh God! Oh God!" he would moan. I always trailed well behind George and Dennis. As I neared George, he would leap from the ground, totally refreshed and sprint another hard 440 followed by several "Oh Gods" mixed with gutteral moans.

I later learned that George was belly-breathing, a method of quickly replenishing oxygen. The moans and prayers were decoys to ward off evil spirits.

George has every anatomical defect he has written about. He has Morton's foot. He has had a heel spur syndrome and plantar fascial strain. He has somewhat tight heel cords and forefoot varus of 6-7 degrees with a hypermobile first ray. When his heel first hits the ground, he rolls excessively over the heel. As the whole foot comes into contact with the ground, the arch lowers excessively. It has to overpronate to lower the inner metatarsal heads to the ground. His plantar fascia is strained by all of this pronation, and it pulls on the heel bone (calcaneus). This pull, over and over again with each foot plant, mile after mile, causes a heel spur. The heel becomes sore and aching. The arch aches.

I made George rigid orthotics out of plastic. His softer, flexible supports were comfortable but had too little support to take care of the heel spur. The new supports worked fine, but as soon as the heel got better, he switched back to the lighter, less effective supports. The heel pain returned and George would switch back to the more rigid supports. We all break the rules, even George Sheehan.

After running, George was rather tight. He felt a good warmdown would keep him flexible. Not so. Peter Stein and I were convinced that stretching was the key. We did the plough, and the static and dynamic heel cord stretches. We stretched our hamstrings. George felt great. The next week he ran a 3:01 at the Trail's End Marathon in Seaside, Ore. This was his personal record at age 56.

George and I have been together often since that week in Hayward. We have learned much from each other, I much more than he. Our friendship is deep—the kind of deepness that follows long runs together in Miami, Atlanta, Seattle, Boston and San Francisco. I am enough of a friend to be on George's mailing list.

FRANK MATSON

Frank Matson, a 43-year-old distance runner, had enjoyed running 60-80 miles per week for the past several years. He was in excellent shape and came to my office in June of 1975, complaining of right heel pain. The pain was at the bottom of the

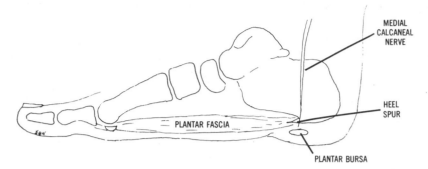

FIGURE 5

Plantar Heel Spur

heel and he'd had this for about a month. It was so painful when he entered my office that he could not run and he even had pain when walking. His past medical history appeared to be unremarkable, and there were no symptoms of gout or arthritis. (Sometimes these problems will cause heel pain and they should always be ruled out with laboratory tests and a complete physical examination.)

My examination of Frank revealed that he had fairly normal foot structure with only two degrees abnormal motion at the rearfoot and 3-5 degrees abnormal motion of the forefoot. He had a mild Morton's-type foot on the left foot, but his right foot appeared to be functioning normally—and this was the painful foot. When he ran, however, his right foot pronated more than when he walked. This pronation appeared to be linked to his painful right heel.

When a patient comes in with fairly normal foot structure, yet still has pain at the bottom of the heel, I begin thinking of a plantar heel spur (*Figure 5*) or plantar fascial strain (*Figure 6*), with or without entrapment of a nerve.

I examined Frank very carefully and found that there was pain in the area of the right heel where the muscles of the foot attach to the heel bone (calcaneus). This is the location of the heel spur. However, there also was pain along the course of the medial calcaneal nerve as it ran beneath the inside ankle bone. This nerve apparently was caught up in a stone bruise, just beyond the area of the heel spur. Frank seemed to have a combination of heel spur with an entrapped nerve, as well as tenderness of the plantar fascia.

The plantar fascia was more tender when the toes were pulled up and pressure was applied on this very tight band of tissue which runs from the toes to the heel. When runners have only a plantar fasciitis, their pain is more severe when running on the balls of their feet. When there is a heel spur problem, the pain appears to be more severe at heel contact. When there is a medial nerve problem or stone bruise, heel contact also causes the problem. Frank, however, had all three.

X-rays of Frank's foot showed there was a very large heel spur. Despite the fact that he had a large heel spur, we decided to treat him conservatively with a combination of mixed corti-

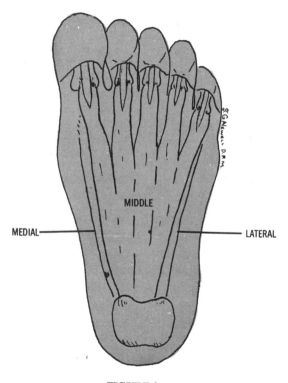

FIGURE 6

Plantar Fasciitis

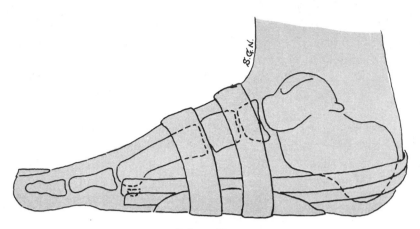

FIGURE 7
Low-Dye Strapping

sone injection into the bursa and heel spur area, rigid plastic orthotics, tape strappings of the foot and ultra-sound physical therapy. The rationale for each treatment is as follows:

• The injections helped break up soft tissue scar formation which might allow the medial calcaneal nerve to work its way free. Also, injections into any bursa or false sac in the area might take care of the problem. The most injections I will give a patient are two or three at weekly intervals. Too much injection may mask the symptoms, and the patient may go out and hurt himself. He must be advised to take it easy for 2-3 days following an injection.

• The orthotics stop abnormal pronation and lessen the pull on the plantar fascia and on the heel spur area. Orthotics take about two weeks to be made, and in the interval I like to use a tape strap to rest the plantar fascia and arch. This is very helpful with heel spur syndrome and plantar fasciitis.

• Ultra-sound causes deep vibration of sound waves which can break up scar tissue, increase circulation and decrease inflammation. It is used most successfully two times a week for 2-3 weeks.

With this combination of conservative treatment, Frank's mileage improved to where he could do six miles a day, but he was unhappy with this. He wished to do eight, nine, 10 or 12 miles a day. I discussed with him the possibility that surgery could make him better, but there was no guarantee. I said I doubted, however, that the surgery could make it any worse.

Frank made his decision when he no longer could run six miles a day and was back down to two or three. Apparently, the orthotics were helping, but the effects of the physical therapy and injections were wearing off.

Surgery was performed in October 1975. At that time, a large heel spur was excised, the plantar fascia was released from the heel spur area and the medial calcaneal nerve entrapment was surgically excised. Frank had a postoperative dressing and a wooden postoperative shoe for two weeks, then the sutures were removed. He gradually returned to running. Six weeks following surgery, he was running three miles a day. After two more weeks, he was up to six miles a day, and by January 1976, his running was unrestricted. He felt that this surgery was completely successful.

Most plantar heel problems respond quite well to conservative measures consisting of plantar strappings, padding and orthotics. Occasionally, cortisone injections are necessary and, at times, treatment for arthritis or gout will work quite well if these conditions are present. Very rarely is surgery required, but in this instance it was indicated and was performed with good results.

LES CARLSON

Les Carlson, a 40-year-old gymnastics instructor, also was active in long-distance running and many other sports. He desperately needed good lower extremity function for his job and recreation.

However, he had complaints of left arch pain and swelling with some discoloration, red and blue, at the area where the muscles of the foot attach to the heel bone. He said he had injured his foot while playing basketball. He had jumped up for a rebound and upon landing had felt a tearing sensation at the bottom of his foot.

About two years earlier, he had strained his right foot in a similar manner, and it had healed on its own. He also had a neuroma on his right foot which was operated upon several years before.

My examination of Les' foot showed a large bulge where the plantar fascia should attach to the heel bone. When I pulled his big toe back towards his head, the plantar fascia did not become tight on the inner edge of the foot, suggesting to me that there must have been a partial rupture of this area. There was swelling and all symptoms of soft-tissue tearing.

My diagnosis was post-traumatic rupture of the medial plantar fascia of the left foot, but I also wanted to rule out the possibility of a stress fracture of the heel bone. X-rays showed none, although it is possible to have a stress fracture which doesn't show up until 6-8 weeks later, when the fracture is healing.

My treatment consisted of a strapping of the left foot (*Figure 7*) and temporary soft supports. I told Les to lay off basketball for the next few weeks while we were evaluating his problem. On his next visit, he noted that the left arch was greatly improved and his soft supports were quite comfortable. He had been using them while playing golf but had not been playing basketball. He had removed the strappings since the tape became somewhat worn after a few days, but he said the taping definitely helped.

At this time, we casted Les for the rigid orthotics to provide for arch support, lessen the pull of the plantar fascia and allow proper healing. I also retaped his foot. Since the soft tissue healing takes 3-4 weeks, I suggested that he wear this type of strapping with weekly changes for the next four weeks.

Les is now playing basketball with his soft supports. I have suggested to him that he always tape his foot prior to basketball to prevent recurrence of his problems, and that he use the plastic supports for distance running and everyday use.

RICK BROWN

Rick Brown is a world-class half-miler, whom I had the pleasure of meeting in November 1973. At that time, Rick was complaining of pains in his right arch. He noticed that the pain came on as he was doing a 10-mile run. He'd never had such trouble in the past but had a history of recurrent achilles tendonitis. He also recalled that he had shin splints at the beginning of track seasons.

I noticed as he was walking that Rick's arch was depressed more than normal. This overpronation did not correct itself at

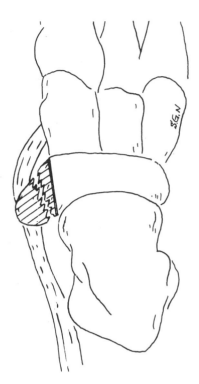

FIGURE 8

Os Navicularis

toe-off, and he had what we call "delayed resupination" of the foot. This basically means that the foot was not becoming a rigid lever at lift-off and that he had an inefficient mechanism for getting his foot off the floor. This wastes energy.

When Rick walked, he externally rotated his feet 7-10 degrees on the right side and 10-12 degrees on the left side. His left leg was a quarter-inch shorter that his right. This means that Rick was externally rotating his left foot for stability, possibly secondary to the short left leg. He had a moderate irritation where the achilles tendons attach to the heel bone and a runner's bump in this area. On his right foot, the talus (ankle) bone was protruding to the inside of the foot, and there was irritation over this area. The arch beneath the talus was, likewise, irritated. There was clawing of very long second and third toes, and an

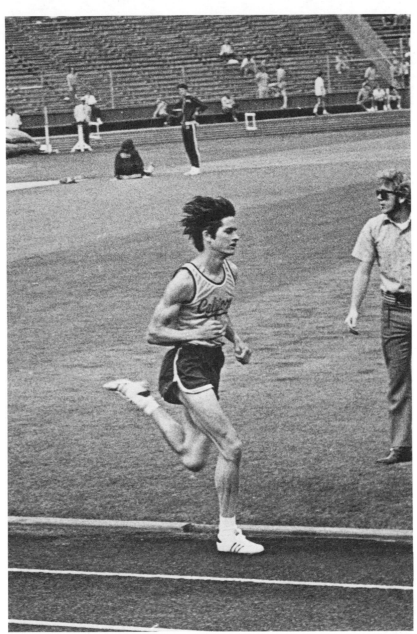

World-class half-miler Rick Brown was treated by Dr. Subotnick for arch problems resulting from overpronation.

obvious Morton's foot syndrome with a short first metatarsal, instability and hypermobility of the first metatarsal.

All of this added up to the pronated foot which lends itself to overuse syndromes and foot strain. Rick's problem was that he had only six degrees of pronation available at his ankle, but all of the deformity he had added up to 10 degrees. This meant that four degrees had to be absorbed elsewhere, even if his foot was going to be as flat as it would normally be. This four degrees was taken up in the ankle and leg, and caused additional strain.

Treatment consisted of soft orthotics. I told Rick to come back for rigid orthotics but somehow lost contact with him for nearly two years. He told me in late 1975 that the soft orthotics appeared to help him, but he was now interested in a more rigid type. I made him a pair of Sporthotics, semirigid supports used for speedwork and racing, and a pair of plastic supports for everyday use and distance training.

He reached the final of the Olympic Trials 800 meters several months later.

DIANNE YOST

Dianne Yost was a college quarter-miler in 1974. She came to me complaining of bumps on the insides of the arches on both feet. Her problem was diagnosed as "os navicularis" (*Figure 8*), which means there was an extra bone in the arch area.

The type of running Dianne did, interval running, caused the bone to rub on the inside of the shoe. Because the bone was protruding so much it was necessary to surgically excise it and to remove the posterior tibial tendon somewhat to the bottom of the foot. This resulted in a higher arched foot. The surgery was successful. The moral is that lumps and bumps in the feet which cause a lot of problems can usually be treated fairly well surgically.

16

Heel and Achilles

JOE HENDERSON

Joe Henderson is a hobbit. He is always happy. He is always smiling. I have never heard him say an ill word about anyone. He is almost too good to be true. Joe has been one of the leaders in influencing hundreds if not thousands of people to run sanely, safely and gently, and as far as I am concerned he is a primary mover in preventive medicine with his approach.

Joe came to me several years ago with a very painful "runner's bump" on his heel (*Figure 1*). The ailment is technically a retro-calcaneal exostosis, a painful blister or bursa (fluid-filled sac) on the outside of the heel alongside where the achilles tendon attaches to the heel bone (calcaneus). As the heel bone rolls against the counter of the shoe, there is irritation. This irritation first causes a blister, and later the body tries to protect the skin from further blistering and forms a bump. This is usually painful. The bone reacts to the pressure by forming more bone, and as more bone is formed the spur at the back of the heel presses on the skin and causes even more pain. Eventually, the achilles tendon is stretched over the bone spur and there is irritation and inflammation. When this happens, there is a full-blown, very painful runner's bump on the heel.

This is about what Joe had. He had a biomechanical deformity which caused him to place excessive stress on the outside of his heel during contact. Due to this, he wore down the outside of his heel more on one side than the other. The side with excessive wear was the side with the painful bump. He would land on the outside of his heel and quickly roll in (pronate) because of the imbalance in his foot. This caused the sequence of events as described above.

Not all patients I have seen with the retrocalcaneal exostosis have such a sequence of events. Some runners actually are born with a bony shelf on their heel which needs only the rocking action of their heel during running to cause serious damage to the achilles tendon and soft tissue which lies above the bump. Other runners have such a high arch or high pitch to the calcaneus that this causes a rather normal-appearing heel to tilt backwards and, again, rub into the achilles tendon during the rigorous action of running.

Generally, however, it appears that landing on the outside of the heel and then rolling inward is the cause of the injury. This was hurting Joe to such a point that he was using his own rather sensible, conservative treatment measures. He was cutting out the back of his shoe. This is a good idea. In fact, we have suggested to some runners to cut out the heel counter and apply elastic to hold the shoe together, and in this way relieve the pressure over their heels. This sometimes helps, but not always. We also suggest that conservative or non-surgical treatment should utilize some type of heel lift to stop the heel from having pressure in the counter of the shoe. Also, the patient should have a good orthotic with a rearfoot post or heel control device so there is not so much rolling in of the calcaneus or heel at heel contact.

The problem with injuries is that those caught early tend to respond very well to the foot supports. Those which have lingered on and on before treatment is sought tend to form more scar tissue, which is rather unyielding and does not respond as well to conservative measures such as arch supports, cortisone injections, icing, ultra-sound and various oral medications which slow down inflammation.

We tried all of these conservative measures with Joe, but it appeared that his deformity was too long-standing to respond well. He had what we call rearfoot varus along with forefoot varus. He pronated excessively and needed orthotics to balance up his feet. Despite the orthotics, he still had the deformity, and

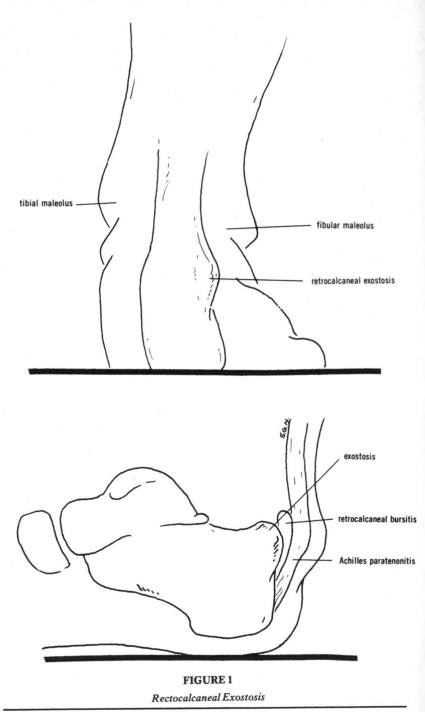

tibial maleolus

fibular maleolus

retrocalcaneal exostosis

S.G.N.

exostosis

retrocalcaneal bursitis

Achilles paratenonitis

FIGURE 1

Rectocalcaneal Exostosis

The Running Foot Doctor

the bony shelf would not go away on its own. We took x-rays, and both of us agreed that it was time to remove this bony shelf.

I recall that day that Joe came to the hospital, put on his green surgical suit and marched into the operating room shaking like a leaf. He had decided that it would be best for him to stay awake throughout this procedure, so we used local anesthesia. I gave him a bit of medicine to calm him down, and then numbed up the back of his heel with local anesthetic. I recall Joe talking to the doctor who was monitoring his vital signs (blood pressure and pulse) while I knocked off the bump on the back of his heel with a bone-cutting instrument. The surgery itself took about 30-40 minutes and appeared to be completely successful.

Following surgery, I placed Joe in a cast for 2-3 weeks. I recall telling him that the cast would protect his foot and leg, and that he could go ahead and do reasonable exercise following the surgery. Joe came in for a cast check one week after the surgery, and his cast was almost totally gone on the bottom. I learned that he had been walking a mile a day with his cast on to keep in shape. He also was riding his bike daily. As long as he had the cast, he really could do no harm and I told him the exercise was a good idea.

Since I have operated on Joe, I have had countless patients with heel bumps. Most of them have responded well to conservative treatment, consisting of stretching, balancing the foot with foot orthotics, icing and staying off the hills until the inflammation had gone down. I still have some patients with significant deformity who need the surgery. By and large, it is successful, and the runners return to painfree exercise as Joe Henderson has.

KEN WILLIAMS

Ken Williams is a long-distance runner in his 30s. In 1975, he won the 30-mile Levi Ride and Tie Contest, despite the fact that he was unable to do any fast training. He came to my office that October complaining of bilateral tendonitis of the achilles He noted that he'd had this problem for the past four years and had been unable to run well for prolonged periods. Previous treatment had consisted of rigid orthotics made two years earlier. He said they were not working since his achilles tendon still hurt. The only trauma he'd had was a right ankle fracture 10

---

years before. The rest of his medical history appeared to be normal.

Ken told me that he was running from 70-110 miles a week when he began having pain along the tendons of the Achilles. The pain was so severe that he quit running for three months. Since that time, he had been going through periods when the achilles tendons became better with the rest and immediately became painful again when he returned to running, especially when doing speed work or running on the ball of his foot. He was quite discouraged.

My examination showed that he had thickening of the sheath of the achilles tendon. We call this "tenosynovitis." This had been present for four years and had not responded to rest or other conservative treatment, including orthotics. It was apparent to me that further conservative treatment probably would not do much good, and that he would either have to be content being a long, slow distance runner utilizing heel lifts and supports or consider changing his sport to biking or swimming.

Another alternative was that he subject himself to what is considered to be experimental surgery. The surgery is somewhat controversial and entails a surgical release or sectioning of the sheath of the achilles tendon (*Figure 2*). The achilles tendons in cases like Ken's are completely normal, but the covering of the tendon which is similar to the skin on a hot dog or sausage, is thickened, tight and swollen. This sheath is placing pressure upon the tendon which moves within the sheath. It appears as though the sheath can be damaged by overuse injury, excessive speeds or strain which might occur when running hills.

Most patients with this problem respond quite well to rest, icing, stretching and orthotics. In fact, only about one-half of one percent of the patients ever will need surgical repair of their achilles tendon sheaths. Dr. Gabe Mirkin suggests that some patients with this problem may have a high uric acid level, which we call "gout," and he has noted that patients with an even mildly elevated uric acid respond well to treatment of the gouty condition.

I agree with Dr. Mirkin and have had similar experiences with three or four of my patients with this problem. Ken Williams did not have gout, however. He had done some reading and thinking

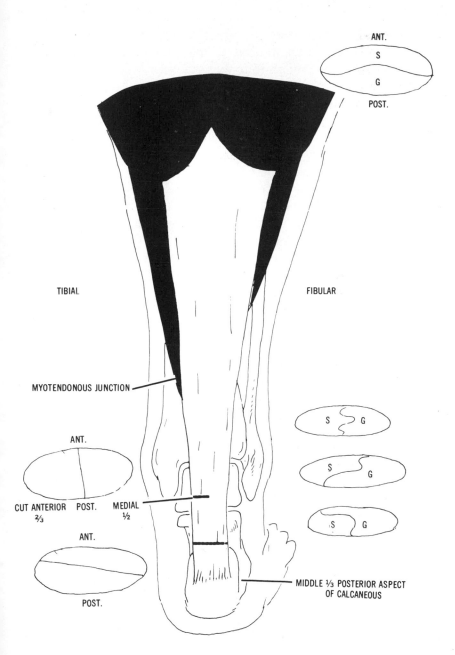

FIGURE 2

Achilles Tendon Lengthening

about having surgery prior to coming to my office and was fairly well convinced that he wanted to have the surgical procedure since he had been through four years of other treatment with no success.

I examined Ken thoroughly, and came to the conclusion that surgery would probably be the logical step since he did not want any of the other alternatives as suggested above. The sheaths were thickened and were painful. Even though he had rested, they would not get much better.

Ken had surgery in November 1975 under general anesthesia. An incision was made at the back of each foot and leg, and the achilles tendon sheath was found to be swollen and adherent to underlying fatty tissue and the tendon itself. It was abnormal in appearance and did not appear to allow the tendon to glide well. Abnormally thick tissue was excised and tight, constrictive tissue was released surgically. The tendons appeared to be completely normal. They were not thickened nor damaged. It was only the sheath of the tendons that appeared damaged.

Ken was placed in casts for two weeks. Following this, we started intensive physical therapy with ultra-sound and stretching over ice. He recovered quickly enough to compete in the Ride and Tie race in June 1976. Ken called to tell me that his surgery was completely successful, that he was able to run fast and train fast, and that he was very pleased at having it done.

I must admit that this is still controversial surgery and that not all authorities agree on its usefulness, but in my experience with about a dozen patients, all have been apparently satisfied with the results. One of them, Jack Browne, ran a personal best in the mile after his surgery. Results of other surgeries are likewise encouraging.

17

Ankle Sprains

TREATING SPRAINS

The most common ankle problem is the sprain. Sprains are partial or complete tears or ruptures of ligaments. Ligaments' main job is to prevent exxessive *normal* motion, whereas tendons' job appears to be preventing abnormal motions.

Therefore, it is normal to invert the foot, but excessive inversion leads to tearing of the ligaments on the outside of the ankle joint—the "inversion sprain." Likewise, it is normal to pronate the foot, but excessive pronation may cause a deltoid ligament or inner ankle ligament tear.

Ligaments have special sensory mechanisms in them which are supposed to tell your body if you are moving the joint to extremes of motion. Thus, when you begin to turn your ankle, you are warned that damage may take place and you shift your weight to the other foot to avoid a sprain. The problem is that, following a severe sprain, these kinesthetic sensations are disrupted. The only way that they become normal is through proper rehabilitative exercises.

When the pain has diminished, practice hopping up and down on the involved ankle. Also, strengthen the peroneal muscles on the outside of the ankle. This is done by holding a door and then pressing the door with the outside of the foot, placing tension in the peroneal muscle groups. Flexibility in an ankle that has been sprained is maintained by doing circles with the foot, starting with small circles and making them larger. When running can be done comfortably, run straight at first and then progress to wide figure-eights which progressively become smaller.

Sprains come in degrees. A "first-degree sprain" is recognizable because there is very little swelling or damage done to the ligaments, and there is mostly just tenderness with pressure over the ligament. There may also be tenderness with extreme fast running, but generally the athlete can walk without a limp, do raises on the balls of the feet without problems and jump up and down on the balls of the feet. Usually, following one of these sprains, ice is utilized. The ankle is examined to see if it is stable. The athlete might be taped and allowed to return to practice or competition. These sprains usually take care of themselves within three days.

A "second-degree sprain" usually has more tearing of the ligaments, often the anterior lateral colateral ligament. The athlete walks with a very mild limp, but has discomfort and tenderness when raising off the heels, and definitely has pain when jumping on the balls of the feet. This injury responds well to icing, and with proper taping the second-degree sprain is converted to a first-degree sprain and the athlete can return to running. It is necessary to take the ankle prior to any vigorous activity on irregular surfaces to prevent respraining. This especially holds true for rough cross-country courses.

"Third-degree sprains" are the serious ones. There is a limp and pain with walking. The athlete has a great deal of pain when raising off his heel, and can't jump up and down on the ball of the injured foot. He should not be allowed to return to vigorous activity, and the ankle should be examined carefully to rule out fracture or complete rupture of a ligament.

Treatment usually consists of elevation, ice and crutches. If the third degree ankles are severe enough, the athlete might need a cast for three weeks, following by taping. Crutches are used until the athlete can walk without pain.

A "fourth-degree sprain" is severe. It is an unstable sprain in which the anterior lateral colateral ligament is completely ruptured. If this sprain is not treated properly, it will lead to an unstable ankle which chronically gives out and may lead to arthritis or spurring in the front of the ankle.

These sprains show instability upon examination and should

be x-rayed to rule out fracture. Then a cast is applied for 4-6 weeks or immediate surgery is perfomed to repair the ruptured ligaments.

The best time to examine an ankle is during the first 20 minutes following injury. There is less spasm and swelling at this time, and one can feel the ligaments and see if they are torn or partially torn. Likewise, it is easier to see if the ankle is stable or unstable. As this time elapses, more swelling takes place and it is more difficult to evaluate the ankle.

One of the problems with the acute ankle sprain is a fracture of the talar dome on the inside of the ankle joint. Such fractures often are not detected until 6-8 weeks after the sprain. In fact, radiographically they sometimes are not evident for six months following the sprain. If you have had a bad sprain which appears to have healed on the outside of the ankle but there is still some pain inside the ankle joint itself, you should be x-rayed again to rule out one of these chip fractures.

CURTIS SELLS

Curtis Sells, a 16-year-old high school student, visited my office in August 1975. He was one of the outstanding jumpers and hurdlers during track in his area. He had damaged his right ankle five years earlier, and he also noted that his left ankle had been injured. Curtis noted that there was now so much pain in the front of his ankles that it was very difficult for him to compete in cross-country or do any jumping event.

When Curtis walked up and down the halls of my office, there was an audible popping sound at the front of the ankle. He said this painful popping had made it impossible for him to do any running or jumping for the past two months. Past treatment had consisted of prolonged rest, but when he resumed activity the popping returned and pain in the front of the ankle returned.

My examination of Curtis showed that he had extremely flat feet with excessive pronation. He had tightness of both achilles tendons. There was pain at the front of both ankle joints, and there was readily detectable spurring at the front of the ankle when I examined this area with my fingertips (*Figure 1*). There was pain associated with pressure over the spurs and the tendons over the spurs were inflamed because of the pressure of

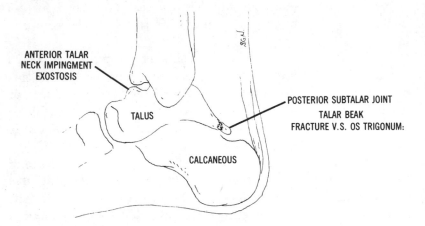

ANTERIOR TALAR
NECK IMPINGMENT
EXOSTOSIS

TALUS

CALCANEOUS

POSTERIOR SUBTALAR JOINT
TALAR BEAK
FRACTURE V.S. OS TRIGONUM:

FIGURE 1

Impingement Exostosis of the Ankle

the bone itself. When Curtis had his foot flexed upward, bone hit bone at the ankle joint area, which appeared to be causing the spurs. I am sure that jumping activities might also have aggravated this, but, more likely, his past history of injury and repeated ankle sprains contributed to the problem. Tightness in the achilles tendon was probably secondary to the limited motion at the front of the ankle joint. The snapping noise of the tendons probably was due to their moving over the abnormal spurs at the front of the ankle.

The normal, conservative treatment for this problem consisted of foot orthotics to control abnormal foot motions, and stretching exercises for the achilles. In addition, Curtis had enough inflammation that he was given injections of cortisone solution. X-rays were take, both in the relaxed and stressed positions, to determine the amount of spurring taking place.

Curtis returned to the office a couple of weeks later, noting that his ankles were somewhat improved, but when we reviewed the x-rays it was noted that excessive spurring was taking place and that this was limiting the motion at his ankle joints. Further examination also revealed a crunchy sensation, which demonstrated some overuse arthritis at the front of the ankle joints where the bone spur of the foot was hitting the bone spur of the ankle.

Curtis was operated on in October 1975. Large spurs were removed from adjacent aspects of the foot and ankle. We noted a thickening of the joint capsule over the spurs, with inflammation present, and that the tendons themselves were inflamed as a result of the spurs.

Curtis was placed in below-the-knee walking casts, on both legs. When the casts were removed, he started stretching and strengthening exercises. By the next track season, he was able to compete well.

Another patient came to my office recently and told me that his main concern was in beating Curtis at the high jump. He also had spurring at the front of the ankle, very similar to what Curtis has, and had undergone surgery for this problem. This made me think that some sports, such as jumping, have hazards which can result in spurring at the front of the ankle. I have also noted that football linemen have a crunching between the foot and ankle which, again, results in spurring. Hurdlers can get this problem from repeating jumping and hitting the hurdles, as can basketball players from repeating jumping. It appears as though bone forcefully hitting bone can cause spur formation as the body tries to limit excessive motion to decrease the strain on soft tissue surrounding a joint.

Curtis Sells' story is not unusual. He responded well to the surgical approach when conservative treatment failed. I am still left with the thought, however, that some sports, with all the good they produce, may have inherent hazards as well. It is my job, as well as the job of others in sports medicine, to investigate these hazards and what we might do to prevent them.

BILL JENSEN

Bill Jensen had twisted his right knee in the 1973 Bay-to-Breakers race. He then went ahead to injure himself in a later race, where he fell and twisted his right ankle on the very hilly course. Along with these complaints, he had pain at the bottom of his right heel.

When I examined his right heel, there appeared to be a rather firm mass that I could delineate with my fingertips.

Biomechanically, Bill had the type of structure which allowed him to place a lot of stress to the outside of both heels and then roll in. He had what we call rearfoot varus, 4-5 degrees, and a great amount of bowleggedness. He had six degrees of forefoot varus or imbalance. His flexibility appeared to be fairly good.

X-rays were taken and showed no heel spur. My initial impression was that Bill had a new growth under the skin in the subcutaneous fat of the right heel. Treatment consisted of an injection into this mass to break up what felt like hard scar tissue and allow the tissue to return to a more normal state. I used cortisone for this, because it has a softening effect. I also used a medicine called Wydase, which tends to spread fluid and remove a bursa.

Bill was given a strap, which he could put on and take off the foot. This would help build up the arch. I placed felt on the insides of both shoe heels. Bill returned a few weeks later and reported that the right heel did not hurt, but now his right knee hurt. He also had a new complaint, a plantar wart. We took care of the wart by trimming and applying acid solution. He was given some padding with a strapping of his foot.

He came back in October, complaining of pain in the front of the ankle joint. Examination revealed a spur, which may have been caused by his frequent ankle sprains.

Bill was pleased with the effect of felt in the shoes and thought he would try this rather than go to a soft, flexible orthotic or to the more rigid orthotic.

Since then, I have seen Bill at several races. He reports that he is doing well with various adjustments of his shoes, using felt padding in the heels and under the arch. He has learned to care for his own foot problems.

18

Shin Splints

JO ELLEN HOWARD

Jo Ellen Howard drove several hundred miles to see me, and I was sorry that she had to travel this far to get help. A runner on the Linfield College track team, she complained of recurring pain in both legs. She thought it was some form of shin splints. She said, as she was getting into peak condition, the pain would begin and would reduce the amount of time she could spend training. Because of this, she was unable to set any outstanding marks in the half-mile and mile because she just could not do the type of training necessary.

Jo Ellen had seen several other doctors who had taken x-rays and ruled out any fractures of the bone or stress reaction of bone. It appeared that she had a pure overuse running injury with no systemic manifestations. My examination showed that she had good rearfoot structure but about four degrees of forefoot varus. This is not an unusual amount. Her tibia was bowed about five degrees. When she walked her feet were straight ahead. She pronated approximately eight degrees from her neutral position. This, in itself, is only mildly excessive.

Upon examining Jo Ellen, I found that she was extremely tender in the lower one-third of both legs, to the inside of the shin bone. This is where the posterior tibial muscle is. When she made her arch high by using this muscle, there was more tenderness, and when pressing over the muscle there was extreme tenderness. There was also some swelling present.

My diagnosis was "posterior tibial myositis" or, more simply, inner leg shin splints. This appeared to result from the fact that when she ran her feet pronated, pulling excessively on these tendons. Jo Ellen would have no problem at all while walking or hiking. Her feet are fairly good. When she runs, however, there appears to be enough stress to cause trouble.

Treatment consisted of making her a good pair of soft orthotics for speedwork and competition and rigid orthotics for distance training and everyday use. She went on a program of Vitamin E, 1000 units daily for two weeks, to be cut down eventually to 500 units a day and later 250 units a day. She also took Vitamin C, 1000 milligrams a day, and responded quite well to this combination of treatments.

PAT MOORE

Pat Moore, a 28-year-old distance runner and wife of Dan Moore, a 2:30s marathoner, first saw me in March 1975. She had shin splints as well as bunions which did not bother her but were of concern. She'd had similar pain a year earlier, but it had gone away by itself when she rested.

My examination revealed that the flexor muscles of both legs were inflamed. These are the muscles which move the toes up and down. It is possible that she was trying to toe off too much, or that she just had imbalances in her foot which caused a problem. My biomechanical examination showed she had extremely flat feet with 9-10 degrees of forefoot varus and two degrees of rearfoot varus.

I suggested to Pat that orthotics would help with the shin splint problem, since as her arch was depressed when she excessively pronated it pulled on the tendons. I also suggested that she would need some good physical therapy, ultra-sound in the office and ice at home to reduce inflammation.

The bunions appeared to be the type which should be watched and not operated upon. They could possibly improve, or at least not get worse, with the functional plastic foot supports.

Pat started from no running the week she came to see me, went to 15 minutes a day the next week, then 20 minutes a day the following week, then 25 minutes a day. Within six weeks of her first visit, she was completely asymptomatic. She has not had any problem since then.

GOUGH REINHARDT

When I first saw Gough Reinhardt, he was 45 years old and had many sub-three-hour marathons to his credit. He was bothered by a shin splint syndrome over the posterior tibial muscle area, the muscle mass in the lower one-third of the inside of the leg. This type of pain usually is caused by abnormal foot pronation during running. Gough noticed for the past three months he had progressive stiffness and pain. His mileage now was severely limited, and this was affecting his racing.

My diagnosis was "posterior tibial myositis" with swelling within the tendon sheath and belly. I was concerned about the amount of swelling and gave Gough an injection of Xylocaine, a local anesthetic, mixed with Wydase, a medication which disperses swelling. X-rays were taken to make sure there was no underlying stress fracture and to evaluate the bony configuration of his feet.

Biomechanically, he had one degree of varus in the rearfoot and 5-6 degrees of instability in the forefoot. His flexibility at the ankle joint was somewhat limited.

I instructed him on proper flexibility exercises for his tight posterior muscles and told him he could run with felt heel lifts but to decrease his mileage to 2-3 miles day.

Two weeks later, Gough received rigid orthotics. He was still sore enough to require another injection, this time with cortisone added. I did this because of a grating sensation over the muscle when the foot was moved up and down, a sign of a very tight tendon sheath which is in need of some anti-inflammatory medication.

After a week of running 2-3 miles a day with the new orthotics, Gough noted that his feet did not seem to be as flexible as he would like them to be in the orthotics. I suggested that he might need softer orthotics for running faster, but that the rigid orthotics should work well for everyday walking and slower distance running. His posterior tibial tendonitis was greatly improving and he was running a 7-8-minute pace.

Two weeks later, on May 3, he was up to four miles a day. The tendonitis was greatly improved. After several more weeks, he returned to the office requesting racing orthotics. He was given softer orthotics with slight heel lifts. He also was complaining of some strain of both achilles tendons, and I noted that his flexibility was a bit decreased.

More than a year later, Gough came back to the office with a rather advanced achilles tendon strain on both legs. This was at the junction of the tendon to the muscle belly. He said that he had been stretching before and after running, and that his mileage was at 150-200 miles a month. He'd actually cut his mileage in half, yet this didn't help with the achilles tendonitis much. He complained that he could not get up on his toes or run fast because of the pain in the backs of his legs.

My examination revealed that the achilles tendons were three times their normal size and were very tender. The strength was normal, and there appeared to be no ruptures, indicating that the inflammation was only of the tendon sheath. He was given cortisone injections into the sheath of both achilles tendons, and the rearfoot posts of his orthotics were improved upon to decrease pronation. He was told not to run for the next 48 hours, to elevate his feet and to stretch over ice before and after running. He returned two weeks later, greatly improved. The right achilles was now only two times normal size, and the left one was 1 1/2 times normal size. He was running with only mild pain, though he was still very tender to the touch. I instructed him to continue stretching over ice, limit his mileage and run slowly.

Within two more weeks, Gough was up to 50-60 miles a week, his left achilles was normal sized and the right was only slightly larger than normal. He was running without pain. Despite the fact that he was doing flexibility exercises, he still appeared to need felt heel lifts on top of his orthotics to raise his heels between an eighth- and a quarter-inch.

When I saw Gough again some months later, he said his achilles were fine but that he had pain beneath the right heel. My examination revealed that he had what appeared to be a stone bruise-type plantar neuroma. This was treated with an injection of cortisone to break up adhesions around the nerve. He was told to return if his pain resumed, but Gough has not had to come back to the office since 1975.

BARBARA WAYNE

Barbara Wayne is the wife of Ron Wayne, a national champion

in the marathon. She would like to be active in jogging, but every time she goes more than two or three miles she has extreme tightness in the back of her legs. This tightness persists and she has some swelling and even walking becomes difficult.

My examination showed only mild to moderate instability of her feet. I could find nothing wrong in the back of her legs. Yet I had her run and the tightness appeared in the back of the legs. I concluded that she was having a functional tightness of the muscles, which we call a "functional compartment syndrome." I suggested that physical therapy and orthotics might do some good. The soft supports made her feet comfortable. She was able to run farther, but she still had cramping.

I appears that Barbara is one of those rare individuals who just is not cut out for running. Every time she runs, she has swelling of her muscles inside the very tight sheath which surrounds the muscle. This causes pressure on the muscle and pain. The only real treatment for this is a surgical procedure where the sheath of the muscle is excised. We only would consider this in people who *must* run. Since Barbara could substitute other sports such as riding a bike or swim, she rejected the surgery.

19

Runner's Knee

CYNDY POOR

Cyndy Poor was a member of the 1976 US Olympic team in the 1500-meter run. I saw Cyndy in 1975 when she was part of an experimental group to decide exactly what foot supports and felt in the shoes would do for runners. At that time, she had some complaints of left knee pain and some left foot pain. I noted that she had a bunion on the left foot.

I made soft supports for her and took x-rays. The bunion on the left foot had an inflamed capsule, so she was given an injection into the capsule to ease the inflammation. She called me a month later, saying her foot was not bothering her anymore and the left knee was much better.

Evaluating Cyndy biomechanically, we have found that she had fairly good structure. Her rearfoot was almost perfect and her forefoot only showed 3-4 degrees of imbalance. She had a great deal of tightness in the muscles in the back of her legs which probably was secondary to running on the balls of her feet and not doing proper stretching exercises afterwards. I told her about this, and since that time she has been doing more stretching.

Movies of Cyndy running showed that she has a very powerful stride, yet tends to "cross over" somewhat, placing her feet from one side to the other rather than in straight line projection. This is rather common in women runners, because of their wide pelvis, which causes their feet to angulate inward from the hip joints. The bunion on her left foot is the result of her jamming this joint

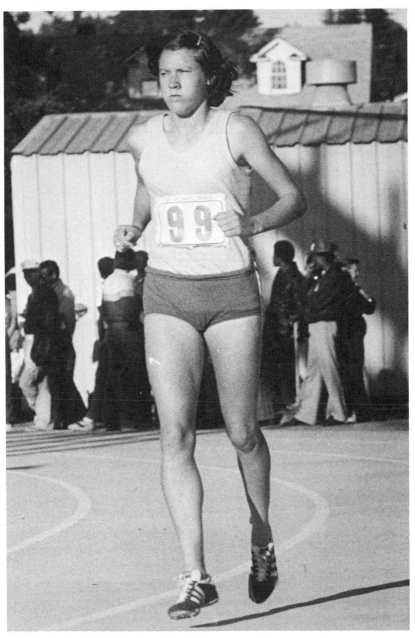

Jeff Johnson

Former "runner's knee" victim Cyndy Poor qualified for the 1976 Olympic team in the 800 and 1500 meters.

and causing some bony reaction. An orthotic may be helpful for this.

Despite the fact that Cyndy appeared to function well without orthotics in the motion-analyzing movie, she functioned even better with felt inside the shoes and better yet with the soft orthotics. Since she is a half-miler and miler, she was advised to use only felt or a soft orthotic during competition.

HANS TEMPLEMAN

I saw Hans Templeman, a college distance runner, in June 1974, at which time he had multiple running complaints: left heel bruise with a bursa on the heel which pops out with running, knee trouble on both sides (more so on the left) and shin splints on both legs.

My examination revealed that his pelvis was level and that the knee had good strength, but the attachment of the patellar tendon (the tendon at the undersurface of the knee cap) formed a somewhat oblique angle and that, when he forcefully used the thigh muscles to stabilize the knee cap, it had a tendency to move towards the outside of the leg. We call this "lateral sub-luxation" of the patella (*Figure 1*), or a mild form of "chondro-malacia" of the knee (*Figure 2*). Chondromalacia is a softening of the cartilage of the undersurface of the kneecap as it moves over the thigh bone, the femur.

Hans appeared to have chondromalacia and perhaps a little bursitis in both knees. There are many bursae around the knee joint and sometimes they become inflamed. He had rather large bony prominences on the femur bones which were just his anatomical characteristics, but they appeared to be causing some tendonitis in the hamstring area.

Examination of the feet showed a moderate amount of in-stability with 5-6 degrees of forefoot varus (instability in the forefoot) and 2-3 degrees of rearfoot varus instability. He had a tendency to throw his left foot out when he walked and ran. The hips, however, were normal in rotation.

X-rays were taken of the feet and showed a classic case of Morton's feet with very long second toes and metatarsals, and short, somewhat excessively mobile first metatarsals. This, of course, placed undue stress upon his foot and leg.

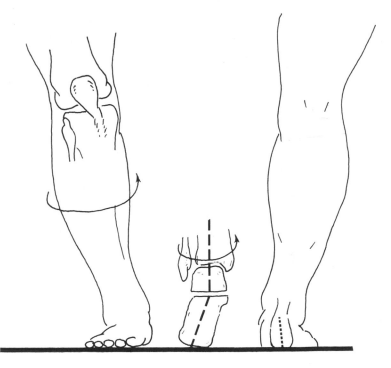

FIGURE 1

Lateral Patellar Subluxation

Further examination indicated that Hans had a fairly high arch when the foot was off the ground but, it was depressed upon weight-bearing. This suggested a need for some form of orthotic to stabilize the arch. When Hans was walking, as his feet flattened, his legs internally rotated, and this added to the instability of the kneecaps.

I made orthotics for Hans and put him on straight leg raises to build up the quadriceps muscles which support the patella. I had him raise his legs and forcefully contract the muscles in the front of the thigh, holding them to a count of 20, and do at least 20 of these daily. I also had him do some stretching exercises.

When he received his orthotics, they decreased the unnecessary rotation taking place in the leg because of the Morton's foot. The knees became asymptomatic and caused him no problems whatsoever in later running. The only problem Hans

---

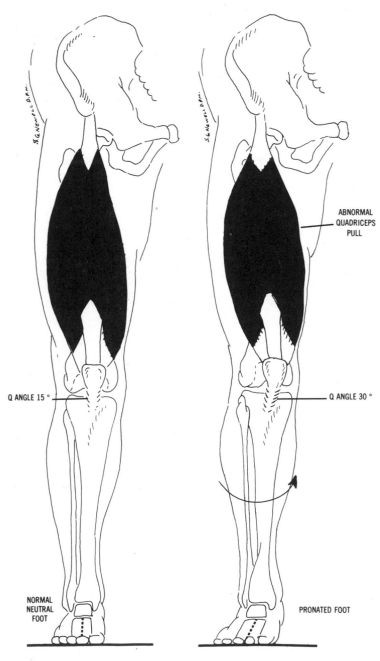

Q ANGLE 15 °

NORMAL NEUTRAL FOOT

ABNORMAL QUADRICEPS PULL

Q ANGLE 30 °

PRONATED FOOT

FIGURE 2

Chondromalacia of the Knee

had was some blistering with the orthotics, which is not unusual. This was corrected quite easily by shaving the plastic down and putting some Spenco material on top of the supports.

DONNA VALAITIS

Donna Valaitis was trying out for the Canadian Olympic team in 1976 and had been training strenuously. She had complained of pain in the arches, off and on, for the past two years. She also had pain in the knees under the kneecaps, which could have been caused by increased mileage in her training. She had been training 70 miles per week. Finally, she had some left hip pain.

My examination revealed that Donna had internal rotation of her legs with secondary strain at the outside of her knees and some tightness of the iliotibial bands. She had a tendency towards what we call "lateral subluxation" of the patella. As she ran, taking long strides, the kneecap had a tendency to go toward the outside with resulting rubbing of the cartilage on the under surface of the kneecap. Donna had a high-arched, rigid foot, with some wobbling of the rearfoot. Apparently, this was enough to cause some knee instability.

Treatment consisted of orthotics and relief was immediate. The rearfoot post controlled her heel contact. Her knee arch and hip pain went away. While she just missed the Olympic team, she enjoyed her best season of running ever.

20

Hip and Low Back

JIM HOWELL

When I first saw Jim Howell several years ago, he had noted progressive stiffness in his back to the point where he could no longer run and had difficulty even walking comfortably. He was so stiff he had trouble bending forward. He had seen other medical professionals, and opinions were volunteered as to the possibility of arthritis or some back abnormality which might need future surgery. Despite all this, no one had ever really looked at his feet or ascertained whether or not he had a limb-length discrepancy (*Figure 1*).

Jim's feet were rather interesting, too. They weren't pronated. They actually had an arch that was too high. We call this a "cavus foot." One foot functioned differently from the other, and one leg was longer than the other. He had a tilt of his pelvis, and the belt line on one side was lower than the other. This indicated that one leg was longer than the other.

I told Jim that he might have some form of sciatica, which could have been associated with a short leg. It was possible that he had some form of arthritis, but this seemed unlikely. I thought he may have had some serious malformation in his back or a disc problem. His back wasn't really tender, however.

When I laid him on his back and had him raise his legs up, there was a small amount of shooting pain going down the back of one leg, but the other leg appeared to move up fine. (This is a test for sciatica to see if stretching the nerve running down the

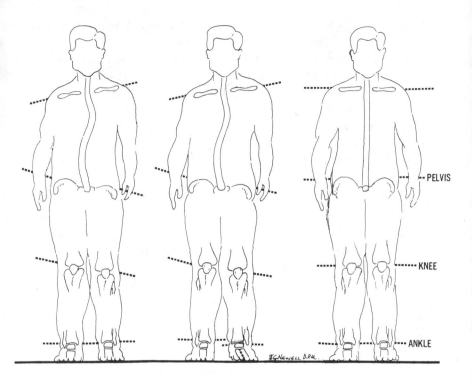

FIGURE 1

*Anatomical Short Leg (left), Functional Short Leg (Center),
Disappearance of Functional Short Leg with Orthotic Control (right).*

back of the leg causes pain.) Yet Jim's tendon reflexes and neurological reflexes were all normal. The indications were that the limb-length discrepancy was causing his problems.

I decided that it wouldn't hurt to balance up Jim's feet with some form of foot orthotic incorporating a heel lift to make the pelvis level, and also to put him on flexibility exercises for the tightness that he had accumulated from his sore back, legs and thighs. Jim's feet were casted and some of the highness in the arch was taken out in the cast to allow his feet to be a bit more flexible. He was given a heel lift to compensate for short-leg deformity which was in part due to the short leg itself and in part due to one foot functioning a bit more pronated than the other, even though both had extremely high arches. A high-arched foot doesn't absorb shock well and needs to be balanced up somewhat differently than a low-arched foot.

Well, to make a long story short and long treatment course even shorter, Jim went from a non-runner back to the great athlete that he was before all this trouble began. (He had run in the Olympic Marathon Trail in 1972.) His flexibility increased. His pain went away, and he became a normally functioning individual. This is an example of how a biomechanical approach might help someone with pain in the low back as well as in the legs or feet.

JOHN ANDERSON

John Anderson is a well-known East San Francisco Bay runner in his 40s. His wife, Ruth, is a well-known international distance runner, an age group record-holder in the marathon. I look forward to seeing both of them at running events.

I have spent many races trying to pass Ruth. I have studied her running style from arear. I have analyzed movies of Ruth's running gait. Ruth rarely has running injuries. She is slender and has an economical stride. Her feet are extremely pigeon-toed (adducted), and her heel pronates excessively at contact. She has a short heel and foot contact, and rolls of her forefoot at toe-off. Her toe-off, like most runners', is actually a *lift*-off. Her foot rolls over her toes and her momentum carries her body forward as her foot leaves the surface. She actually crosses her feet over and toes in on the hills. Because of this her knees are stable. She has a stable, efficient uphill running form. She uses a short stride with no excessive knee lift. Orthotics or foot supports probably would hinder Ruth. They would cause her to be even more pigeon-toed, and she would trip over her feet. Besides, she doesn't get hurt.

Ruth's husband, John, is another matter. I recall receiving a phone call from John in 1974. Two and a half weeks earlier, he had pulled his left hip while running with his wife. He was 46 years old and a veteran runner. Ruth was quite unhappy because he was having trouble sleeping and walking and was starting to get on her nerves because he couldn't run.

He told me, when he came to my office, that he'd had surgery several years before, resulting in a fusion of the low back. He noted that he had a similar pain in his hip approximately one year before, but it wasn't as severe and it went away on its own. He also complained of pain beneath the second metatarsal heads and numbness of the feet. There was no history of arthritis.

I examined Dr. Anderson (he's a veterinarian), and came to the conclusion that he had a short right leg (*Figure 1*). Because of the shortness in that leg the right pelvis was lower. He also happened to pronate his right foot more than his left foot. Looking at his shoes, the right one had more excessive wear than the left. He had a curvature of the spine and pain over the left sacroiliac joint. Some of the shortness of the right leg appeared to be secondary to spasm and some appeared to be due to the over-pronation of the right leg.

Further evaluation of John showed that the joint beneath the ankle, the subtalar joint, had fairly good motion and no abnor-malites. The ankle joint also had good motion. He had Morton's feet with long second metatarsals and a rather short excessively mobile first metatarsal. This was more so on the right side.

John was a basket case. He had trouble walking and bending. He could not bend over past the level of his knees, let alone touch the floor with his hands. He was uncomfortable sleeping and desperately wanted to return to running, but this was totally out of the question.

Soft orthotics were made to balance up the shortness which had occurred, and the pelvis appeared to be level. John was told to start walking, and to do bent-knee situps as well as stretching exercises. He returned a month after his first visit and reported that the numbness on the bottom of his feet was getting better. He felt almost ready to run. He had been walking a mile every other day, doing his situps and could now bend over past the level of his knees.

It was at this time that we casted him for the permanent plastic orthotics, and these were made over an actual plaster of paris mold of his feet. They were then balanced up to hold his heel perpendicular to the ground. When John had no orthotics at all, his heel was rolled in 6-7 degrees or more on the right side.

By the time his rigid orthotics were dispensed, he already was nearly asymptomatic with the soft orthotics which were helping to rotate both beet in. Within two weeks, he was running up to five miles a day in the rigid supports. He was sleeping comfortably. He was able to stretch and almost touch the floor with his fingertips. The supports appeared to rotate both feet inward so that they were both pointing almost straight ahead. They allowed him to pronate mildly to moderately, but he did not have the excessive pronation that he had without the supports.

John Anderson's case helped me realize how much podiatric sports medicine can do for some patients. Here was an example of a patient who had a problem that clearly did not appear to be the type normally treated by a podiatrist. John had low-back and sacroiliac pain. He had done some reading on his own and had convinced me that, if I balanced up his lower extremities with orthotics, his low-back pain should go away. John was so sincere in his concern and so determined to go back to running that I felt I should at least try all of my theories out on him to see if what I had been preaching actually would work. It did work and I am glad that we went along with the treatment plan.

Certainly, not all patients who come to me with running injuries such as low-back pain are helped with orthotics. Many of them are referred to orthopedic surgeons because they have true pathology in the low back which only an orthopedic surgeon can treat properly. There are, however, some patients with low-back pain, due to limb-length discrepancy and overpronation of one foot or the other, who benefit greatly from orthotics. It is these patients I hope to help.

part IV

ON YOUR FEET

21

Young Feet

A child who wants to run should not be discouraged from doing it, but on the other hand a child who has no interest in running should not be pushed by his parents. Children normally play hard enough so that no organized sport is necessary until they reach school age.

Most children enjoy sports. However, I have known some children who do not, because of the aching they get in their legs. These often are overuse syndromes which may be corrected easily with some type of foot orthotic. Younger children tend to do well in a soft, inexpensive, flexible support. We use these because their weight is such that the softer materials will still support their foot, and because they outgrow supports so rapidly that it is a financial burden on the parents to have to provide their children with more expensive supports every time shoe size changes. I try not to use a rigid support for a child until he weighs more or until I am fairly certain that bone growth has stopped. (Bone growth stops anywhere from between the ages of 14 and 16 in a woman and 15 and 17 in a man.)

What complaints do I notice most in children who are running? The younger children who are going through growth spurts between the ages of eight and 12 tend to have problems at the attachment of the achilles tendon. We call this "apophysitis." The leg bones appear to grow faster than the tendons. The posterior tendons or the achilles tendon is placed on a stretch, and it pulls at its attachment to the heel bone. There is a second center of ossification here, and it becomes inflamed. Treatment is a felt heel lift and reassurance to the parents that the child will outgrow this problem and may continue to run, as long as the pain is not bothering him significantly.

Another form of apophysitis is Osgood-Schlautter's disease This is simply an irritation of the attachment of the patellar tendon between the kneecap and the front surface of the leg. There is often enlargement and inflammation of this bony process, called the "anterior tibial tubercle." Children usually outgrow this deformity, too, though they go through quite a bit of discomfort during their early teens when they have this problem.

We have been somewhat successful with treating Osgood-Schlautter's disease by using foot orthotics to slow down transverse plane rotations in the leg, and with wetsuit material knee braces to help hold the kneecap in place. If the pain is really bothering the runner, he should be told to wait out the season and choose another sport in the meantime. He should also be reassured that he will probably outgrow this problem.

Children also may have heel problems when they are doing a lot of jumping. They may even develop bursitis or something which mimics a heel neuroma. We utilize a soft orthotic with a felt heel as well as physical therapy for these problems and generally have good success. We have at times had to resort to an injection of a very small amount of soluble cortisone for a bursa problem in younger children. However, I tend to treat their problems on a functional basis and shy away from any medicines if possible.

Parents often ask me if their children's feet are developing normally or if there is something they should be doing in the way of exercise or foot supports. They also want to know how much foot deformity is inherited.

I feel that a great deal of the instability of the feet is inherited. Parents with bunions, shin splints, arch problems or Morton's foot syndrome may pass on these tendencies to their children. When we have the opportunity to examine babies as they begin bearing weight and walking, we often can suggest various types of exercises that the parents can do with the children, or supports or braces which, when used when the child is young enough, quickly correct soft-tissue problems and make a child's growth much more normal.

I like to treat with some form of in-shoe device any child whose feet appear to toe-in, toe-out or pronate abnormally. What this does is allow the foot to correct its own deformities. This protects the child while he is growing and, hopefully, allows for more normal development of the foot and lower extremity.

We, as a population, tend to overreact to foot and leg problems in the very young child. (This was most apparent with my own three children.) When a child starts to walk, he has a tendency to externally rotate his feet for stability. We note this same phenomenon in older persons. This gives a wide base from which to function. Externally rotated feet have a tendency to appear flatter or more pronated. Also, a child may have a tendency to sleep with his feet tucked in underneath him, with the weight on the outside of the feet. This causes the in-toed problem. If the child sleeps just the opposite, it may cause an out-toed problem. If one foot is tucked underneath and the other turned out, then there is an inequality of rotation at the hips, and this will be mirrored in the gait pattern. Various straps and bands which can be applied to shoes or to sleepers which will help correct this problem are available.

Flat feet in children, per se, is nothing to be terribly alarmed about, but it should be checked out to make sure that there is no inherent problem. The doctor may tell you that the child will outgrow this, and he may be right. But it is my feeling that the feet should still be protected while the child is outgrowing the deformity.

If there is anything disturbing in the way children walk and run it is always wise to have the checked. Likewise, if there are problems which run in the family the children should be screened early.

22

Running Shoes

Before taking a recent run, I went out to the garage and looked at the 50-odd pairs of shoes I have, inspecting the backs and looking at different wear patterns. I tried to pick out the models I thought would be ideal for training. I was getting ready for a marathon, and I didn't want to get blisters or have a breakdown from the mileage I was doing.

It occurred to me then that every shoe has its own individual characteristics and that every shoe must be right for someone, although none may be right for everyone. Finding the right shoe takes time, trial and error. You have to shop around. Your choice depends upon your weight, stride, speed, range of motion in the foot joints and skin type—plus, of course, the shape of your foot and the height of your arch.

What do I think the "ideal shoe" should have? I would like a shoe for training which has a thick sole, 2-3 layers of rubber material. This rubber should be firm on the portion which contacts the surface, yet somewhat spongy in the next layer to allow sheering forces between the middle layer and the one next to the shoe. The third layer should be firmer.

The types of sole available now are the waffle, ripple and the standard crepe. The waffle sole appears to absorb some transverse plane stresses, yet to allow contact stress absorption the material must be somewhat soft and it wears out rather quickly. These are great soles for running hills and dirt courses, and are comfortable on cement as long as the nubs of the waffle hold up. The ripple sole also helps absorb contact stresses, but there are problems on courses with small rocks or mud, which are picked up in the ripple sole itself. Crepe soles are the most common and generally wear the best. They do not have the grasping or gripping power of the waffle and ripple soles, yet they are more practical for everyday use on cement in regard to durability and being able to repair them.

The sole should be somewhat beveled at the rear to decrease the lever arm. This helps with shin splints and with those who are overstriders. A beveled heel also is beneficial in downhill running because everyone has a tendency to overstride and to brake with the heels while running down hills.

Heel height is a problem. We have found that the negative-heel shoe (heel lower than the forefoot) is not good for running, though it appears to be a good exercise device. I have been wearing negative-heel shoes for several years, off and on, and find them best for standing or for use immediately after long runs. However, I am uncomfortable on long walks with my negative-heel shoes.

It appears that some form of heel lift is necessary for running to ease some of the stress on the posterior muscles and achilles tendons. This also appears to give a mechanical advantage, causing the body weight to be forced forward along with the center of gravity. The ideal height of a running shoe heel is open to debate. The higher the heel, the less stress on the achilles, yet less force comes from the achilles when it is supported.

The ideal thickness of the sole under the forefoot is another debatable point. Too much thickness causes a strain of the achilles. Not enough thickness causes pain under the metatarsal heads. There must be enough flexibility to allow for a "break" or easy bending at toe-off, yet the shoes also must give forefoot protection.

As for materials, I like a firm leather heel counter that will support and grasp the heel well. It should be high enough so that when an orthotic is worn the height of the orthotic will not cause the heel to slip up and down in the shoe. It should be strong enough to help decelerate deforming forces at heel contact. Uppers of nylon appear to be good for most runners, although leather uppers may offer more stability. Runners in colder climates with a lot of rain and snow may want all-leather shoes which can be waterproofed. Leather also has the advantage that shoe-stretching materials or hot water can be placed on it and, as the shoe is worn, it stretches out over bony prominences.

What can you tell by looking at the bottoms of your shoes? Those who tend to contact on the outside of their heel obviously will wear their shoes down fastest in that area. It is normal to contact 2-4 degrees to the outside of the heel. Runners should be concerned about outside heel wear only if it is far to the outside of the shoe.

Those who contact well back on the heel are overstriding and have a wear pattern at the back and center of the heel. Runners with extreme pronation of the feet will contact on the inside of the heel. They are candidates for orthotics even before they have experienced foot and leg trouble because they are putting grossly abnormal stresses on themselves. Likewise, people who run on the balls of their feet tend to give biomechanical deformity hints. Rigid, cavus-type feet wear more to the outside of the sole, while pronated feet wear more to the inside of the sole. Shoes which are too tight often have abnormal wear under the toes.

When buying shoes, look at them on a table. The bisection of the heel should be perpendicular to the ground. As the shoe begins to wear or deform, again check this to make sure it is somewhere near perpendicular. When gross deviations occur due to faulty manufacturing or abnormal wear, the shoe should be discarded. Perhaps you may need a shoe which is more rigid in the heel counter area and has a wider or "flared" heel.

Also look at the thickness of the soles on both shoes. You can find up to a quarter-inch discrepancy between shoes. Such a manufacturing defect was pointed out to me recently by a patient who complained of a right foot problem. Not coincidentally, her right shoe was a quarter-inch lower in the heel than the left.

How good are the arches in shoes? Motion-analyzing photography has shown that, by and large, the arches really aren't "arch supports" at all. They are just soft sponge rubber which feels good but offers no biomechanical control. It is impossible to build an arch into a shoe which is right for all people, since feet differ so markedly. Any attempt to make such an arch would meet with failure because only 5-10% of wearers would be comfortable with it. The rest of the people actually would have more problems rather than relief.

Ideally, if one is having foot and leg troubles, he should get a custom-made arch which can be transferred from shoe to shoe.

23

Other Sports

BASKETBALL

Basketball players tend to be in good shape because they are running forward, backward and side to side. They have well developed muscles and flexibility. Their main problem is that from rebounding and jumping up and down on hard surfaces. This causes jumper's knee, chondromalacia of the patella and jumper's ankle. They also have the problem of spraining an ankle when coming down on the inside of their foot or landing on someone else's foot. Basketball players should have their ankles taped before every practice and game to prevent these sprains.

Early in the season, many basketball players get shin splints in the front of the legs from the hard surfaces. These usually respond to proper stretching and strengthening exercises. At times, foot supports with cushioning under the metatarsal heads help this problem.

The heel spur syndrome is common in basketball players, as is arch strain. A heel spur syndrome responds quite well to Low-dye strapping with felt pads and should be followed up with a semi-flexible foot support to be used during a basketball game. I cover the orthotic with shock-absorbing materials.

Some of the professional basketball players I have treated have dislocated metatarsal phalangeal joints and very bad bunions and hammertoes. Also, they have problems under metatarsal heads. These are treated symptomatically. I try to avoid operating on the athletes until their competitive years are over.

I have had fairly good success in treating jumper's knee and chondromalacia of the knee with semi-rigid orthotics. In some instances, even better results are obtained with a wet suit material knee brace.

BIKING

Bikers are rather interesting inasmuch as some of their pains in the hips and knees appear to be related to the angle at which the foot is inserted into the cleats on the peddles. Generally, the more in-toed the biker is, the less problems he has. Too much in-toeing, however, causes lateral knee and ankle strain.

Bikers appear to do best with a softer support going all the way under the toes. This is because most pressure is applied to the pedal from the metatarsal phalangeal joints or balls of the foot to the end of the toes. Bikers do strange things with these supports, building up the outside or inside in order to suit their symptoms. Whatever they do, if it works, is fine by me. I usually make a soft support for the biker and give them all the supplies necessary to make their own adjustments.

Bikers also get problems between the toes. We attribute this to pressure on the interdigital nerves, causing Morton's neuromas. These neuromas often are symptomatic only when riding long distances, but tend to recur. I have had success in surgically excising the neuromas when symptoms warrant it.

HIGH JUMP

High jumping, in fact all jumping sports, have injuries peculiar to the activity. One of those is the possibility of a sprain when coming down on an ankle which is turned to the inside. People who have a lot of bowleggedness, tibial varum or rearfoot varus, are more prone to these sprains.

There also are problems with overstriding on the approach. I see this in high jumpers who stretch way out before planting one foot and then taking off. This causes anterior shin splints.

Jumpers tend to have very tight hamstrings, but this does not necessarily mean the hamstrings are strong. They should concentrate on strength and flexibility of their hamstrings.

Foot problems in jumpers include plantar fascial strain, heel spur syndrome and first metatarsal phalangeal joint pain. I treat these with soft orthotics and Low-dye strappings.

GYMNASTICS

Gymnastics is similar to dancing. The injuries are frequent and very difficult to treat. Many muscle strains are secondary to rapid movement, and these respond only to rest and then proper stretching and strengthening exercises. Shin splint syndromes are not uncommon. They may respond to taping of the feet or making removable dancer's straps. Knee pain and arch pain respond to similar types of approaches.

The main problem is that many of these athletes have so much flexibility and pronation of the feet, and when doing their exercises barefooted and landing on their feet from the apparatus, injuries may develop. Some types of taping must be carried out.

TENNIS AND RACQUETBALL

These sports have problems stemming from rapid acceleration and deceleration on very hard surfaces. Everyone has heard of tennis toe, which is an inflammation of the first metatarsal phalangeal joint caused by serving and rolling over the toe. It is somewhat similar to golfer's toe which occurs on the left great toe in right-handed golfers.

We treat this problem by utilizing tape splinting and, if there is quite a bit of inflammation, appropriate anti-inflammatory medications. At times, a semi-flexible orthotic is helpful.

These racquet sports also cause trauma to the heel with heel bruises, plantar fasciitis and heel spur syndrome. Competitive tennis players tend to have a lot of knee problems as well as posterior muscle group shin splints. It is just because they need much more arch support than they are getting in the commercial tennis shoes. These problems respond dramatically to proper functional orthotics, either rigid or semi-rigid.

Tennis players usually don't stretch properly and often get some iliotibial band tightness as well as tightness of the achilles and groin. Proper stretching exercises make a big difference.

GOLF

Golfers have problems from walking on irregular surfaces and from following through too vigorously during their swing. They often get an aching in the forward foot, first metatarsal phalangeal joint and may have neuroma syndromes as well as plantar fascial strains. They appear to do well in a semi-rigid orthotic which allows them some flexibility, since they must pronate their feet when teeing off yet need more support when walking on grass.

SKIING

Skiers really have problems when there are structural deformities of the lower extremity. Those skiers who happen to have a tibial varum much over six or seven degrees just can't turn in the direction of their deformity. They use up all of their pronation just to get their foot on the ground when there is a lot of rearfoot varus or bow-legged deformity, and there is no pronation left to set the ski's edge. These skiers have a tendency to hop a lot and are catching edges frequently. They also have a tendency to over-rotate when turning.

With the newer short skis, many skiers have knee pain from riding the bumps. This apparently is from overstraining but may be aggravated by biomechanical problems.

We have had amazingly good success using semi-rigid and rigid orthotics in ski boots for foot problems, as well as cants or wedges between the boot and the ski for leg problems. The main complication is finding the proper boot to fit the various types of feet, and allowing enough room in this boot for some type of foot control.

HIKING

Hikers and backpackers are a very dedicated bunch, similar to runners. These enthusiasts have a myriad of problems which appear to be related to going downhill on loose soil as well as going uphill or on level surfaces on irregular terrain. Their knees are a particular trouble spot on the downhill stretches because of the extra jarring. We have had good results using semi-rigid orthotics which allow some pronation needed for irregular surfaces yet give enough control to take care of the overuse syndromes.

RACE WALKING

Race walkers are interesting to study because they tell us a lot about overuse injuries. They almost never have knee problems because their knees are always extended, whereas runners have knee problems because they are often flexed. The flexed knee position is unstable and lends to knee injury.

Race walkers contact well back on the heel, and have pain in the hip joints and at the front of the legs because they are over-striding and overstressing their antigravity muscles. They also may have problems with one foot being more externally rotated or internally rotated than the other foot. Generally, the use of foot supports lines the feet up in a straight-ahead direction, cuts down on overuse injuries and allows them to train at longer distances without pain.

SWIMMING

Swimmers have lower extremity problems associated with the way they kick. The whip kick, which is the breast stroke kick, is notorious for bothering the knees as well as causing strain at the outside of the ankles. The flutter kick, which is the kick used in the freestyle, is extremely relaxing and seems to cause no problems. It greatly helps runners with tight muscles; after a long run, I often will hop in a swimming pool and just kick for 15 minutes to get the soreness out of my legs.

24

Getting Well

When coming back after an injury, there are a few rules one should know and follow. The first, is that for every day you are away from running or a workout, you lose three days of training. This applies not only to those who are performing at high levels of training or competition but also is applicable to the everyday jogger and runner.

How important is this? Let me illustrate. I had a patient who required surgery for a large extra bone at the inside of his arch. required surgery for a large extra bone at the inside of his arch. We call this an "os navicularis." He began running realize how out of shape he was. He had a myriad of small aches, pains and injuries associated with the plantar fascia and the posterior tibial tendon. He just had not allowed himself the opportunity to take it easy and return to training gradually. I impressed upon him the fact that coming back from surgery is like coming back from an injury. One must not try to run through pain, but run up to the point of pain and then stop.

Another patient had a shin splint problem in the front of the leg. He had a very tight calf muscle which needed stretching, and he tended to overstride. He had to lay off of any heavy running for 2-3 weeks because of his injury. When he returned, he came back full blast despite my warning to take it easy. Promptly, he came down with a rather severe injury in his foot, which turned out to be a shin fracture. Subsequently, I have reviewed the literature on stress fractures and found that bone has a tendency

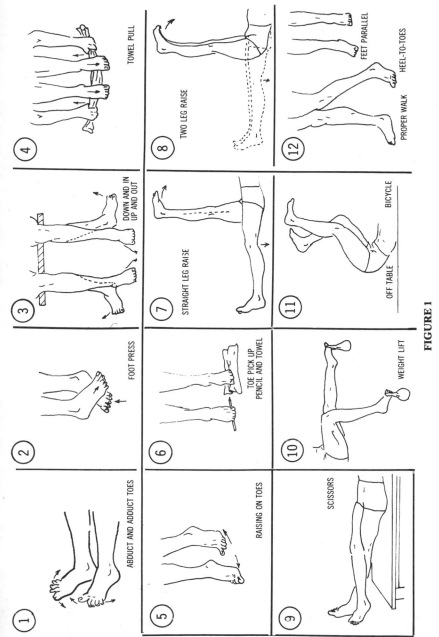

FIGURE 1

Exercises for Feet and Legs

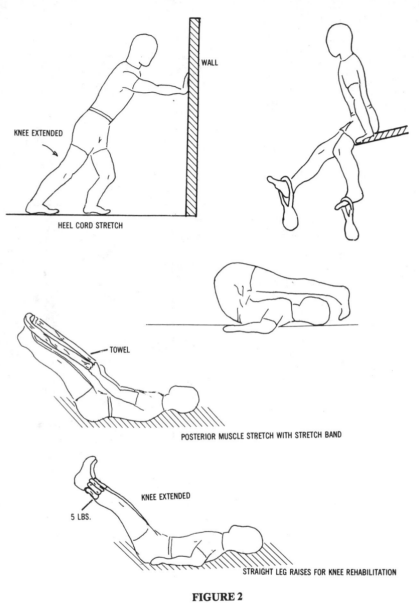

FIGURE 2

Strength and Flexibility Exercises

The Running Foot Doctor

to lose its strength after a layoff of 2-3 weeks making it more susceptible to stress fractures.

I caution everyone who has had an injury which has laid them up for much over two weeks to take it really easy when returning to running. The body adapts to stress rapidly and becomes desensitized to stress rapidly.

I generally tell recovering runners to start with a maximum of 15 minutes a day for the first week at slow paces and to rest one to two days a week. The second week, they may go 20 minutes a day, the third week, 25. In other words, the workouts are increased by five-minute increments per week, and at least one day must be spent resting.

My basic rule is that when the runner can do long, slow distance running up to 45-50 minutes a day, it is then okay to speed up the pace and perhaps even throw in some intervals. From then on, the athlete is on his own.

I do not like to see athletes try to run through pain. If you begin a run with stiffness and pain, and as you run it loosens up, then it is perfectly okay to continue running. If as you run, however, the problem becomes worse, then you are only hurting yourself. You should stop, seek proper medical attention and not run until the situation is reversed. Likewise, I am not so sure it is important to finish every race. If you notice you are severely damaging your body during a race, due to musculo-skeletal pain, I think it is wise to stop.

The most important thing in returning from an injury is common sense. Take it easy, and allow your body to adapt gradually to stress. This, after all, is all that training is.

25

Patients and Patience

George Sheehan has remarked that 50% of what we know will be proven wrong or obsolete. The problem is choosing which 50%. Medicine is still an art. Sports medicine is art, witchcraft, science and trial-and-error.

I have had days when everything goes perfectly—all patients are happy. The combined approach of science (biomechanics), medicine (making the diagnosis and treating properly) and art (reassuring the athlete, and building a mutual trust and respect) works. I have the patience to listen to all complaints and histories, review years of training schedules, examine carefully and treat with concern and skill.

The runner with low-back pain and a short leg was helped with orthotics, heel lifts, and bent-knee situps and stretching. The tight lateral thigh muscle and hip bursitis got better with stretching and orthotics, although I told the runner that my success rate is about 60%. Even the neuromas (aching between the toes) responded to one cortisone injection and foot orthotics.

All surgeries look great—healing well, no unusual pain, good position of toes, no infections. Patient flow is perfect: no long waits for patients, no lulls for me, no emergencies which put me behind, a variety of complaints, interesting people who test my knowledge and who I should be able to help.

Maybe what I do works. Maybe I am helping someone. I feel good.

Then the frustrations set in. My morning hospital surgery is delayed by an emergency appendectomy. My case is unusually difficult. The surgical repair is tedious yet successful.

I arrive at the office 45 minutes late. My patients are unhappy at my tardiness. I am somehow overbooked. Three runners from Nevada stop by to be seen. They can't make it another day. The general practitioner down the road has two patients with infected feet who must be seen. Another fell in a swimming pool, and the post-operative dressing and cast are a mess.

The new patients who called two weeks ago for appointments and have looked forward to relating their problems to me in a relaxed atmosphere have second thoughts about having come. And everyone has a complaint.

"Your orthotics completely cured my knee pain, my feet are great, but I have shin splints—must be the orthotics." I examine the patient and there is extreme tenderness along both shins. Why? I check the orthotics. They hold the arch well. I check for rearfoot control. Perhaps too much. Perhaps this patient needs to roll more on contact.

The patient has been running more with the orthotics because of lack of foot and knee pain—running faster. The supports, however, are uncomfortable. It becomes clearer: overstriding, too much running too soon, perhaps too much rearfoot control and, most important, too short of a break-in period.

This runner had only worn rigid supports for two weeks, her feet were unaccustomed to the control, and she was using her anterior muscles to hold the foot somewhat off on the support. The muscles became overstressed due to this unaccustomed activity, with resulting overstrain and anterior shin splints.

The next patient I greet is returning after last being seen a year earlier. He had missed his scheduled two-week follow-up visit after having had his orthotics dispensed. His runner's knee had disappeared, but his forefoot hurt whenever he wore his orthotics. The feet only bothered him when he ran fast. He liked to run fast. His knee seemed to be healed, so he stopped wearing the orthotics. The knee pain recurred. This was quickly corrected by the orthotics which eventually hurt the ball of the foot. Finally, he returned with a sore foot. The orthotics are "no good." He had been "ripped off." His foot was "almost crippled."

A 10-second examination revealed that the orthotic was a bit too long. It was adjusted. The patient was instructed to return in two weeks. (He did—no foot or knee pain. "Maybe you aren't a rip-off doctor after all," he said.)

And so the day goes on. People with problems, people who have been waiting too long for their turn, patients who resent the cost of medical care, the waiting and the doctor who doesn't know everything.

It is six o'clock in the evening and my last patient, Frank Haggerty, has come from near Stockton with cheesecake. We all have a bite, relax a little, and then I try to figure out what to do to help Frank.

Frank's heel and arch hurt. I have made three different types of orthotics for Frank (soft, semi-rigid and rigid), injected with cortisone and strapped with tape. I have x-rayed and sprinkled holy water from San Lorenzo Creek on his foot. We have gone through every shoe made, altered his running style, rested, biked and prayed. Nothing I do has a lasting curative effect. I have treated Frank for almost three years, and he still breaks down at least once every three months. It would have been easier if the involved foot had a heel spur. X-rays show that both feet have moderate spurs, yet only one hurts.

Frank has waited an hour and a half to see me. He keeps returning and waiting and bringing cheesecake. I still do not understand how to treat his problem.

It is 6:30. I should have been home by now, eating dinner with my family. The kids can't wait to eat. They have a day's experience to relate to me. My wife seeks an adult to communicate with. They want my total attention.

I arrive home at 6:45, late for dinner. I try to concentrate on the family topics, but tomorrow's surgery and the diabetic who is about to lose his leg are still in the back of my mind. I think of the vociferous minority in my local medical community who, even in this day and age, are discriminating against my profession. They are again trying to create conditions in the hospitals that I use which make working difficult, if not impossible.

Dinner is rushed. I have to make evening rounds at the hospital. I manage to relax enough to talk to Jan and the kids, then drive off to the hospital. I return home at about 9:30, put on my running shoes and head for the open road. I recall Joe

Henderson's words: "I am not going anywhere—just running, from what I know not."

Slowly, I unwind. The miles work. Dennis Tracy joins me at the four-mile mark, and we go four together. We talk of the Olympic Trials and his leg.

I return home to Jan, and she realizes that I am human again. I thank God that most of my days go well, are not so rushed and are more rewarding than today.

In the quiet of the evening, I read, write and reflect. I try to formulate plans to reduce the anxieties of life—mine, my family's and my patients'.

Glossary

—A—

Abduct—toe-out.

Abductor hallucis muscle—the muscle running from the great toe to the arch of the foot. It can be easily strained or sprained with excessive pronation, and is often times part of the problem of heel spur syndrome.

Achilles tendon—the large tendon made up by the blending of three muscles, located in the back of the ankle.

Adduct—toe-in or pigeon-toed.

Ambulation—walking or running.

Anaerobic pace—the running pace causing you to be out of breath. During anaerobic exercise you are using a different form of metabolism than during aerobic or exercise when you are not out of breath.

Anterior—towards the front of the body. The toes are anterior.

Antigravity muscles—those muscles at the front of the leg and foot which slow down the foot as it contacts the surface.

Apophysitis—a condition whereby the growth plate, most commonly around the calcaneus at the back and bottom, is tender. It occurs in the adolescent and preteen years.

Arthritis—a condition of a joint upon which there is inflammation. This can be secondary to overuse injury or may be caused by a systemic or metabolic disease, such as rheumatoid arthritis or gouty arthritis (see rheumatoid and gouty arthritis).

Arthrogram—X-ray of a joint.

Articulate—jointed or segmented.

Asymptomatic—showing no symptoms.

Atavistic—refers to the ape-type foot which was a flat foot with the great toe spread from the second toe, enabling this animal to climb. People who have a tendency to maintain an atavistic great toe have a Morton's foot syndrome with a hypermobile first ray and excessive pronation.

—B—

Bipedal stance—standing on both feet with weight evenly distributed.

Bilateral—two sides; both feet, shins, etc.

Biomechanical approach—the approach used when analyzing motion and the structure, and determining the causes of overuse injuries from patterns of motion.

Biomechanics—the study of the biology of motion and mechanics of motion.

Bromhydrosis—excessive sweating with an accompanying foul smell.

Bunion—an inflammation around the joint where the big toe meets the first metatarsal.

Bursa—a fluid filled sac.

Bursitis—inflammation of a bursa.

—C—

Calcaneus—heel bone.

Callus—thickening of the skin secondary to abnormal sheering and torsion forces which may become extremely painful.

Capsule joint—the sac around a joint which holds the joint fluid.

Capsulitis—the condition of the capsule when it has become inflamed.

Cavus—high-arched.

Clubfoot—the congenital abnormality of the foot wherein the foot fails to outgrow the normal in-uteral position. The foot is twisted.

Congenital—inherited.

Contact—when the foot touches the ground during running or walking. Usually, this takes place on the back of the heel towards the outer margin or on the side of the foot.

Cortex—outer covering of the bone.

Cortisone—an anti-inflammatory preparation. Injections of cortisone should be used with prudence. They are very effective when used properly, but when used improperly can cause damage.

Crepitation—a crunchy sensation in a joint which corresponds to an excessive accummulation of fluid or inflammation or cartilage damage.

Cuneiforms—three bones in the foot.

Cyst—abnormal sac containing liquid or semisolid matter.

—D—

Decompression (surgical)—release of tension or soft tissue constricture by surgery.

Dorsiflex—the term used to signify the foot having its dorsal or anterior surface moved towards the front of the leg. During the dorsiflexion, the achilles tendon is stretched.

—E—

Edema—accumulation of fluid in organs and tissues of the body.

Epidermis—outer layer of skin.

Epiphysis—a portion of the bone which in early life is distinct from the shaft.

Epiphysitis—a condition similar to apophysitis but, it occurs on an epiphysis. An example of epiphysitis is Osgood-Schlautter's disease at the knee. This occurs during adolescence and is usually outgrown.

Equinus—a tightness in the structures of the back of the leg which place more force under the ball of the foot and may cause it to pronate.

Etiology—cause.

Everted—turned outward.

Exostosis— an excess growth of bone.

External rotation—angled to the outside. The big toe rotates away from the midline of the body.

—F—

Femur—the larger bone in the thigh.

Fibroma—a hard, firm overgrowth of tissue in an area. This is often secondary to trauma of running.

Fibrosis—an increase of fibrous tissue.

Fibula—the smaller of the two bones in the lower leg. Located to the outside.

Fibular malleolus—outer ankle bone.

Flexion—the bending or turning of a part.

Flexor tendons—the tendons located just behind the posterior tendon which decelerate forward motion of the foot over the ball of the foot and stabilize the toes. These tendons are used for jumping activities.

Float phase—the phase in running when both feet are off the ground.

Forefoot—the front portion of the foot.

Forefoot valgus—the position of the foot when the metatarsal heads face away from the ground to the outside of the foot. The outer metatarsal heads do not touch the ground.

Forefoot varus—the position of the foot when the midtarsal joint or joint in the middle of the foot is tilted, whereby the outside or lateral portion of the foot is on the ground when the inner portion of the foot is off the ground when the subtalar joint and midtarsal joint are neutral.

Functionally neutral—the position the foot is held in for the best function for an individual runner. This functionally neutral position may not be the true anatomical position of neutral. There is a fine balance between functionally neutral and anatomically neutral.

—G—

Gait analysis—analyzing someone walking and running. The gait is analyzed to find functional biomechanics and how it might be improved upon or corrected.

Gastrocnemius—muscle of the inner calf.

Gout—a disease of the metabolism; primary symptom is inflammation of the joints. This is caused by excess uric acid in the blood.

Gouty arthritis—arthritis secondary to a high uric acid that can be treated easily with medications.

Greater trochanter—a boney projection coming off the outside of the hip.

—H—

Hallux limitus—a jamming of the first metatarsal phalangeal joint or the big toe joint, which may occur secondary to overuse arthritis or injury or poor joint structure. The athlete will find that he slowly loses the motion in the great toe joint and may get a bump at the top of the first metatarsal head.

Hallus valgus—an unstable great toe which may be associated with painful bunion or joint.

Hamstring—tendon running from the buttocks to behind the knee. This tendon aids in flexing the knee and decelerating extension of the knee.

Heel cord—achilles tendon.

Heel counter—the hard portion of a running shoe located at the back of the heel which cups the heel and is usually covered with leather.

Heel cup—a device which cushions the bottom of the heel which may be useful for heel spur syndrome.

Heel lift—a felt padding placed in the heel of the shoe to elevate and pad the heel.

Heel spur syndrome—a catch-all term for pain in the heel which may be secondary to a pulling of the plantar fascia and muscles which have their origin from the heel spur area on the bottom of the calcaneus and insert into the heel. It may also be a form of fasciitis or fascial pull.

Heel wedge—material placed under the heel to invert or evert the heel.

Hematoma—a tumor-like mass produced for an accumulation of coagulated blood in a cavity.

Hyperhydrosis—excessive sweating.

Hyperkeratosis—increased thickness of skin which occurs often times with calluses and increased keratin formation.

Hypermobile—excessive mobility in a foot which fails to be neutral in the middle of midstance and does not become a rigid lever at toe-off.

—I—

Iliopsoas—the muscles in the front of the thigh which become tight during long distance running and can aggravate low back pain.

Iliotibial band—that structure running from the hip to the outside of the knee, which can cause snapping and pain over the greater trochanter of the hip and over the knee itself.

Internal rotation—angled to the inside. The great toe or big toe rotated towards the midline of the body.

Interspace—the area between the metatarsals.

Ischemia—loss of proper blood flow to the skin.

—K—

Keratin—a highly insoluble compound found in horny tissue.

Keratolytic—an agent which helps to soften and reduce excessive callus.

Kinesthetic—perception of self-movement.

—L—

Lateral—towards the outside of the body.

Ligament—a band of fibrous tissue binding related structures together (i.e. bones).

Lipoma—thickening of fat in a specific area.

Longitudinal arch—in older literature, there is described a longitudinal arch which is comprised of the medial and lateral longitudinal arch. The arch of the foot is maintained by the integrity of the subtalar and midtarsal joints and very few people have a perfect longitudinal arch. A perfect longitudinal arch occurs when the subtalar joint and midtarsal joint are neutral in bipedal stance.

—M—

Matrix—cells from which nails grow.

Medial—toward the midline of the body.

Medial calcaneal nerve—the nerve that extends to the heel. It is one of the three branches of the posterior tibial nerve which runs behind the medial malleolus.

Metatarsals—bones in the foot, of which there are five, each with a head, shaft and base.

Metatarsal phalangeal joint—the joint where the metatarsals meet the toes.

Microtrauma—very small trauma or wound; tearing.

Midtarsal joint—the joint which controls the metatarsals. When neutral this joint is fully pronated and locked.

Moleskin—a thick felt usually applied to protect the skin.

Morton's foot—a term which is synonomous with a pronated foot and a short first metatarsal which is hypermobile and allows for pronation. Most people with a Morton's-type foot function as though they had a forefoot varus.

Musculoskeletal—a term used to denote the muscles and the skeleton as a system.

Myositis—inflammation of a muscle.

Myotendonous junction—the point where the tendon joins the muscle.

—N—

Neoplasm—a new growth.

Neuritis—inflammation of a nerve.

Neurolipoma—a combination of a nerve and fat problem which also may be a form of stone bruise.

Neurological—pertaining to the nervous system.

Neutral position—the ideal foot position that one would have if he were to have a perfect lower extremity structure. The integrity of the foot and the bones of the foot are so aligned that support will be maintained by structure alone.

—O—

Orthotic—a device to help maintain a functionally neutral position. It is also called a foot support, but actually a biomechanical orthotic functions differently than a foot support inasmuch as it controls motion rather than just supports the arch.

Os navicularis—a second center of ossification over the normal navicular bone in the foot. There is a bulge over the inner arch of the foot.

Osseous—pertaining to bones.

Ossification—to make like bones; become set.

Overstriding—long stride which causes a runner to land on the back of the heel and therefore causing the foot to slap the surface.

—P—

Palpable—readily detectable.

Patella—the kneecap; a sesamoid bone riding over the front of the knee.

Patellar tendon—a tendon that inserts from the inferior pole, or bottom half of the patella, into the front of the leg or tibial tubercle.

Pathology—relating to, involving or caused by disease.

Pelvis—hip bone.

Periostitis—inflammation of the periosteum or membrane surrounding the bone.

Peroneus brevis—a muscle located at the lateral or outer surface of the fibula.

Peroneal—near the fibula.

Peroneal nerve—often this nerve near the fibula is damaged during a sprained ankle. This nerve runs along the peroneal tendon.

Phasic activity—that activity which occurs during motion.

Plantar—bottom or undersurface.

Plantar fascia—the tight band of muscle beneath the arch of the foot.

Plantar fasciitis—inflammation of the plantar fascia.

Plantarflex—to flex the foot downward. During plantarflexion, the Achilles' tendon is relaxed and the anterior tibial and extensor tendon are stretched.

Post—a mechanical means of limiting motion. A post can be an amount of material applied to the rearfoot or forefoot of foot orthoses to control abnormal foot motion.

Posterior—towards the back portion of the body.

Posterior tibial—behind the tibia.

Posterior tibial tendon—that tendon which runs behind the inner ankle bone and has its main function to decelerate abnormal rotation of the foot and help hold up the arch.

Prognosis—a prediction or conclusion as to the course and end of disease.

Pronate—that motion taking place in the foot which occurs as the arch is lowered and the leg internally rotates. Pronation is synonymous with the foot being an adaptive nonsupportive structure.

—Q—

Quadricep muscle—powerful muscles in the front of the thigh which insert into the superior or upper pole or margin of the patella.

—R—

Range of motion—a process of checking the various motions in a joint to find out how much motion is available, and to determine the neutral and functionally neutral positions.

Rearfoot—the back or posterior portion of the foot.

Resupination—the function that takes place after the middle of the time the foot is on the ground. The foot should be neutral an becoming supinated to become a rigid lever for stable propulsion.

Retrocalcaneal—behind the calcaneus.

Rheumatoid arthritis—a form of arthritis which can be controlled with medications but has a tendency to continue the disease process.

Rupture—a tear of a soft tissue segment such as a ruptured tendon or muscle.

—S—

Sacroiliac joint—the joint in the low back on either side of the vertebral column. It can be affected by abnormal pronation or limb length discrepancy.

Sciatica—a nerve-like stabbing or shooting pain which may become intermittent at first and, later, more constant. This pain is caused by compression, stretching or a condition around the sciatic nerve as it leaves the low back area and travels down the back and inside of the thigh and leg.

Scoleosis—curvature of the spine.

Semi-pronated—not completely pronated or neutral. This position for people who have a true tightness of the Achilles is a good functional position.

Sequella—the long-term effect of any injury or treatment.

Sesamoid bones—in the foot, the sesamoid bones are located beneath the first metatarsal phalangeal joint. These bones provide power and spring during jumping events.

Shaft—portion of the bone that is in the middle.

Shin splint—a catch-all syndrome describing pain either in the front of the leg or on the inner aspect of the leg. Both of which may be overuse injuries or, from faulty running style.

Soleus—the muscle in the back of the calf, beneath the gastrocnemius. The soleus, gastrocnemius and plantarus make up the heel cord.

Spenco—a wetsuit-like material used primarily for cushioning and reducing sheering forces in the shoe.

Sprain—a violent twisting, straining or pulling of a ligament.

Stance phase—where the foot is on the ground.

Stone bruise—the lay term for a neuroma or soft tissue mass on the heel which can, at times, be associated with a medial calcaneal nerve problem.

Strain—the pulling or twisting of a muscle or tendon.

Stress reaction—a reaction from abnormal stress.

Stress X-ray—X-rays taken when a portion of the body is stressed to its maximum to see if the ligaments are intact. Stress X-rays are useful following sprain to detect ligamentous rupture.

Subtalar joint—joint beneath the ankle joint. It accepts transverse plane rotations and works like a universal joint allowing the foot to either pronate or supinate.

Subungual hematoma—blood clot beneath the nail.

Supinate—the phase when the arch becomes higher and more rigid. The opposite of pronate.

Sutures—stitches.

Swing phase—the phase when the foot moves freely through space.

—T—

Tarsal tunnel syndrome—the compression of nerves and vessels underneath the inner ankle bone, secondary to stress.

Tendonitis—inflammation of the tendon and/or tendon sheath, often caused by chronic overuse and/or sudden injury.

Tendo-achilles—achilles tendon.

Tenosynovitis—a condition whereby there is inflammation of the tendon sheath.

Tibial malleolus—inner ankle bone.

Tibial varum—bowleggedness.

Toe-off—when the foot rolls forward over the toes and momemtum carries it off the surface. Also called "lift-off."

Torque—the rotatory force; anything that causes torsion.

Trauma—any injury to the body caused by violence.

—U—

Ultra-sound—a form of physical theraphy which causes deep vibration of sound waves used to cause a break up of scar tissue, increase of circulation and decrease of inflammation.

—V—

Valgus—outward rolling of the feet.

Varus—inward rolling of the feet.

Virus—pathological infective agent. The wart is a patholoma virus which can spread as bacteria.

Verruca—wart.

Index

Functional orthotics—see orthotics

Fungal infections—42

—G—

Gait cycles—19, 20, 25

Garnero, Bob—8

Golder, Evan—42-43

Golf, role of podiatry in—119-120

Gymnastics, role of podiatry in—119

—H—

Haggerty, Frank—128

Hallux valgus—see bunions

Heel bruise—66

Heel injuries—14-15, 32, 72, 80-86

Henderson, Joe—vi, viii-ix, 7, 80-83

Henry, James—44-45

Hills, injuries from running—10-12

Hiking, role of podiatry in—120

Hip injuries—104-108

Hirsch, Ben—45-46

Howard, Jo Ellen—93-94

Howell, Jim—104-106

Hyperhydrosis—42

—I—

Injuries, recovering from—122-125

—J—

Jensen, Bill—91, 92

Jumping, role of podiatry in—118

—K—

Knee injuries—4, 6, 7-8, 14-15, 32, 98-103

—L—

Laris, Tom—51-53

Leg-length discrepancy—105

Low-Dye strapping—see taping

Lualhati, Bob—4

—M—

Matson, Frank—71-75

Miller, Jeffrey—59

Mirkin, Dr. Gabe—84

Moore, Pat—94

Morton, Dr. Dudley—31

Morton's foot—31

Morton's neuroma—see neuroma

Muscle tear—12

Muscle tightness—4, 97

—N—

Nails, toe—41-42

Nerve damage—see neuromas

Neuromas—48-53

Neutral foot—20, 26-29

Newell, Dr. Stan—vi

Normal foot-leg structure—24

—O—

Odor, foot—42

Orthotics—5, 34-35, 38, 67

Osgood-Schlautter's disease—111

Os Navicularis—77

—P—

Pagliano, Dr. John—41

Plantar fascia injuries—32, 38, 73

Plantar verrucae—see warts
Podiatry, frustrations of—126-129
Poor, Cyndy—98-100
Pronation—7, 20, 21

—R—

Raquetball, role of podiatry in—119
Racing, first time—8-9
Rectocalcaneal exostosis—see heel injuries
Reinhardt, Gough—95-96
Rotations of leg—20
Runner's knee—see knee injuries

—S—

Schuster, Dr. Richard—67
Sells, Curtis—89-91
Sgarlato, Dr. Tom—2-3
Sharp, Paulette—48-49
Sheehan, Dr. George—6, 12, 31, 67-71, 126
Shin splints—32, 93-97
Shoes, running—113-116
Skiing, role of podiatry in—4, 120
Skin and nails, problems of—40-43
Sports, general—viii-ix, 117-121
Sprains, ankle—see ankle
Spurs—see heel and ankle injuries
Stein, Peter—7-9, 71
Stress fractures—32, 60-64
Supports, foot—see orthotics

Swearingen, Dr. Henry—2
Swimming, role of podiatry in—121

—T—

Taping—69, 74
Tarsal tunnel syndrome—57
Templeman, Hans—110
Tendonitis—see achilles tendon injuries
Tennis, role of podiatry in—119
Tibaduiza, Domingo—54-56
Tibial varum—29
Tracy, Dennis—13-16, 70
Training methods—14-16

—V—

Valaitis, Donna—103
Vierra, Nancy—vi
Walking—19, 120-121
Warts, foot—42-43
Wayne, Barbara—96-97
White, Betsy—47
Williams, Ken—83-86

—Y—

Yost, Diane—79

About the Author

Since he became a long-distance runner in the early 1970s, an increasing portion of Dr. Steven I. Subotnick's patients have been athletes. He practices in Hayward, Calif., and is an Associate Professor of Biomechanics and Surgery at the California College of Podiatric Medicine in San Francisco.

Dr. Subotnick is a graduate of Lewis and Clark College in Oregon and received his professional training at the California College of Podiatric Medicine. He has served as Executive Secretary of the American Academy of Podiatric Sports Medicine, and is a member of the American Medical Joggers Association. In 1975, he published the book *Podiatric Sports Medicine* (Futura Publishing Co., Mt. Kisco, N.Y.).

Dr. Subotnick, who lives with his wife Jan and their three young children in Hayward, Calif., is a veteran of the Boston Marathon and many other long-distance races.

This book's illustrator, Dr. Stanley G. Newell, is a sports podiatrist practicing in Seattle, Wash.